Chakra selfhealing

by

the Power

of

OM

A practical workbook of
healing and spiritual evolution

Rudra Shivananda

Alight Publications 2013

Chakra selfHealing by the power of OM
By Rudra Shivananda

First Edition Published in December, 2002
Second Edition: November, 2013

Alight Publications
PO Box 930
Union City, CA 94587

http://www.Alightbooks.com

ISBN 1-931833-37-0

Printed in Hong Kong

By the grace of
the immortal
Babaji,

I dedicate this workbook for
the benefit of everyone
striving to realize
their highest potential
right now

CONTENTS

Introduction

Are you on the path to realize your highest potential in this life?

An indispensable tool in the arsenal of our body-mind complex for achieving our highest potential is the set of energy centers called the *chakras* by the yogic scientists of India.

The health of the physical body is greatly enhanced by activating and keeping the *chakras* synchronized with the universal rhythm. The spiritual evolution of our soul is accelerated as we work with the higher vibrations and modes of these spinning "wheels of light."

My hope is that a practical workbook for the self-healing of the *chakras* will be particularly useful for those of you who have:

- Begun to think about a spiritual path, but have not yet found or committed to one that seems right. There is no reason why you should not be able to make some spiritual progress in the meantime. These exercises will strengthen you during your search, without committing you to any religion, faith or path.
- Been practicing the physical postures of Yoga, but would like to experiment with the spiritual dimensions
- Embarked on a specific path, but would like to supplement your current practice with working on your energy centers.

What are the *chakras*? These apparently mysterious spinning wheels of energy called *chakras* are in actuality the basic interfaces between various aspects of our manifestation, as well as our connection to the Universe of Energies. They are the dynamos and transformers which function to keep our various bodies *[yes, we have more than one!]* charged with life-force and prevent the damage of overload and the premature death of depletion. When properly tuned and balanced, they are like the hydroelectric plants which control the flow of water to drive huge generators to supply electrical energy to many parts of the world.

Although many books have been written on and about the *chakras*, the majority fall into one of two categories. The first group is based on the complex traditional descriptions of the *chakras* with little or no explanation on how to utilize all the information provided. The second group are the new-age "discoveries" of chakra pioneers into fantastic, complex and unproven systems, primarily based on psychology. It will be at least a generation or more before the worthwhile and proven paths are separated from those that are not.

It is my hope that this work will fill the need for an experiential, rather then theoretical introduction into the various aspects of the *chakras,* consistent with and based on the proven, and time-honored transmission of the yogic scientists of the snowy mountains.

The first part is a brief introduction into the concepts and models which have been assumed to apply for the duration of the yogic experiment. I've kept this part as short and precise as possible so as not to provide unnecessary distraction.

The second part is the actual 7-step practice. The general format is that each practice is preceded by additional information which should be understood and digested before beginning the practice. Each technique has a method and a result. It will take at least 7 days for the results of each technique to flower even though you will feel their effectiveness with a single performance.

The third part of the course-book will address the question of where to go after completing the course. The adventure has only begun and there are many more dragons to slay on the evolutionary path. I've given short descriptions of some of the more accessible paths for the many different personality types.

I have also included an appendix for additional information on the *chakras*.

Words and books cannot give the experience of reality. The set of exercises offered in this book must be practiced for any effect to occur. A minimum commitment of forty-nine days is required for this spiritual experiment to have the desired effects. This is an introductory series, easily practiced, yet powerful enough to open the door to a higher plane of Being.

There is no replacement for a competent spiritual guide or personal instruction on the puzzling and mysterious journey on which we have embarked since time immemorial. For even higher levels of inner experience, you will find the appropriate path through the light of your inner mentor, and the timely appearance of an external guide. The purpose of this set of Chakra selfHealing is to clear away some of the blockages which are preventing you from hearing the pristine inner guidance.

This guide is dedicated to those of you who feel that there is more to life, more to existence, than what is being presented in the limited world-view and value systems which are foisted on us from cradle to grave.

For those who dream of being able to decipher “the hidden, the secret, the esoteric”, the meaning behind the seemingly meaningless patterns of everyday experience.

For those who want to experience the reality behind the maddening appearances which befuddle our senses.

For those who want to be happy!
For those who expect to be happy!

Yoga is a spiritual journey, an experimental path of many dimensions. It is a great joy to share and spread peace to everyone who is open to receiving the higher teachings of the path. May all beings be happy and healthy. May they all be free from suffering and pain. May they all achieve peace and tranquility.

PART 1

Foundation Concepts

Truth is one
The wise call it by various names
Rig Veda 1.164.46

Basic Premises

A short introduction into the assumptions which form the conceptual model for the selfHealing of the *chakras*.

1. The Five-Body System

We are not just this body which we can see, touch, taste, smell, and hear. The particular yogic model which we will be working with assumes that we all possess five bodies. In addition to the physical body, which we can experience with our five senses, we also have an energy body, which functions with our energy interfaces and stores our basic life-force. A third body is where we store our emotional patterns and the potential energy which function in this mode of our manifestation. The mental body is where our mind functions, and is the storage for our mental patterns and associations, as well as for our mental energies. The fifth body is the causal body which is the seat of our soul and repository of our karmic patterns from the cause and effect relationships which we have set into play. When we die, only the causal body survives and can be reincarnated into a new physical body.

There are many systems which give more or less bodies and use different names for them, but the basic underlying agreement is that we have more than just the visible body of flesh and blood, and need to have exercises which work on those bodies as well.

2. The Chakra System

The model recognizes seven main *chakras* and the self-Healing exercises work with six of them. These *chakras* are not on the physical plane, and cannot be discovered by dissecting the physical body. They exist on the other bodies, and their locations can be correlated with various places on our physical body, which is useful for our purposes. These *chakras* vibrate at different rates and have an optimum relationship with each other. When they become out of synchronization with each other or with the Universal Life force, then disease of the body and mind can occur.

3. Spiritual Evolution

The model assumes that we are undergoing a spiritual evolution, and that this evolution is our primary purpose on this plane of existence. What are we evolving towards? That is shown and demonstrated by the great beings such as a Christ, a Buddha or a Krishna, who have come among us as beacons of light for our evolutionary journey. The premise is that these exercises will help accelerate the normal rate of spiritual evolution. The goal is the awakening of the higher human faculties and transformation in the structure as well as function of the human nervous system, hastening the evolution of humanity and healing of physical, mental and emotional ills.

Our present state is only an intermediate stage, and not the ultimate in humanity's evolution. The suffering in the external world is a mirror of the internal pain and confusion in our consciousness. Only by evolving and healing our internal consciousness will the utopian ideal world of the "golden age" be actualized.

If we can jump over our finite mind we can experience a new dimension of existence, expanding the frontiers of our consciousness and enable the expression of the highest creative energies. In order to achieve this, we must transcend the limitation of the confined mind bounded by the stimuli of the five senses, not by escaping from it, but by achieving our highest potential, and redefining, just as the Einsteinian Universe transcended the Newtonian Universe.

4. Kriya System

The tools provided here are for the development of your highest inherent potential. This self-healing program is for those spiritual aspirants who are householders, still living in this world with their specific duties and responsibilities, the career person seeking higher values in life without abandoning the pursuit of worldly goals. However, there must be a willingness to devote the time and effort to work with the tools before any benefits can be attained. Yoga is a scientific system because its effects are repeatable, but it is also an art, because practice is required.

5. selfHealing

True healing involves healing not only the physical, but also the energetic, emotional and mental aspects, and these energy centers or *chakras* are our contacts with those aspects of our existence. The exercises presented are easy to perform and yet very effective to tune and invigorate the chakras, enhancing vitality and health, and cleansing the negative accumulations in the subtle bodies.

We will now examine in a little more detail, the preceding concepts and models, to understand how they fit together in a coherent and holistic way. This is followed by the basic recommendations and structure of the healing system. The final part of this section is on Self-empowerment, which should be read and practiced before starting the selfHealing program.

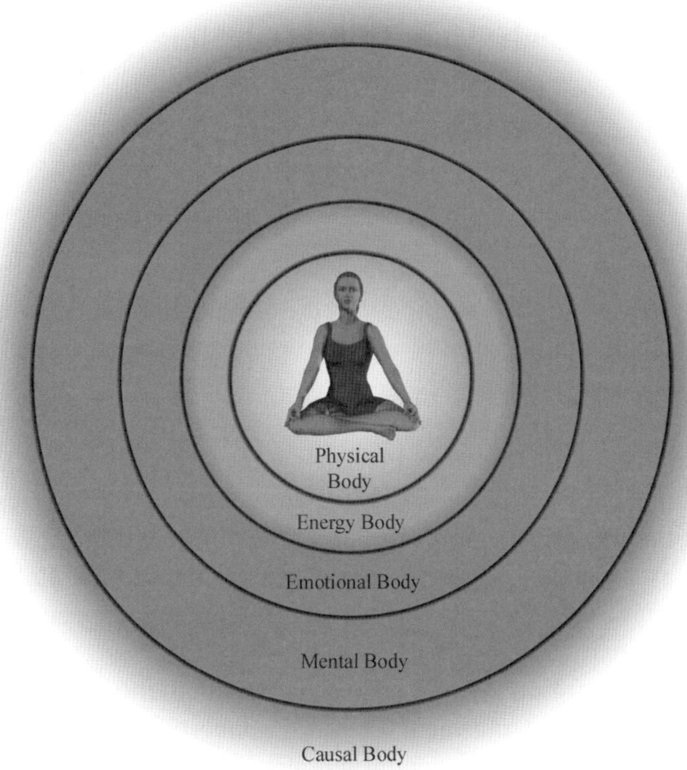

Figure 1 - The Five Body Model

The Five-Body Model for selfHealing

Refer to Figure 1.

1. The physical body is what most of us identify with. It is the only reality which the majority of humanity recognizes, being composed of blood and bones, the nervous system and sense organs.
2. The energy body is just above our normal conscious perception, but can be sensed in recognition of the presence of vitality. It is like an overlay on the physical body energizing and regulating the physical cells. It acts as a channel between the physical world and the higher subtle worlds. Here is where the *chakras* or energy centers are particularly active.
3. The emotional body serves as the mediation between the physical and mental bodies, converting the physical vibrations from the neutral sensations into the "emotionally charged sensations" by adding the qualities of "pleasant" or "unpleasant" or encapsulating it with feelings such as desire or fear. Most physical diseases arise from the emotional or energy bodies.
4. The mental body is the abode of knowledge and analytical thinking. The "emotionally charged sensations" from the emotional body is processed into perceptual units and fitted into patterns calling forth responses which vibrate

back through the emotional body back into the physical realm, causing a physical reaction. This is the realm of thoughts and habit patterns.

5. The causal body is both the home of wisdom and of our *karmic* debts. This is the abode of the evolving soul. Higher abstract and intuitive insights arise from here.

The five-body complex exist and functions in different "dimensions" and each is maintained by a different type of energy, from the physical chemical reactions to the subtlest consciousness energy. Each of the bodies have their own energy centers or chakras as well as energy channels for controlling and distributing of their own level of energy. Orthodox science only recognizes the centers and channels associated with the physical body, where the cardio-vascular system represents the channels, and the brain and various nerve plexuses correspond to the energy centers. As the *chakras* are activated and awakened, you will become aware of the corresponding dimension of reality, giving you a fuller understanding of the lower dimensions.

The tools given here provide a systematic method of awakening the *chakras* safely.

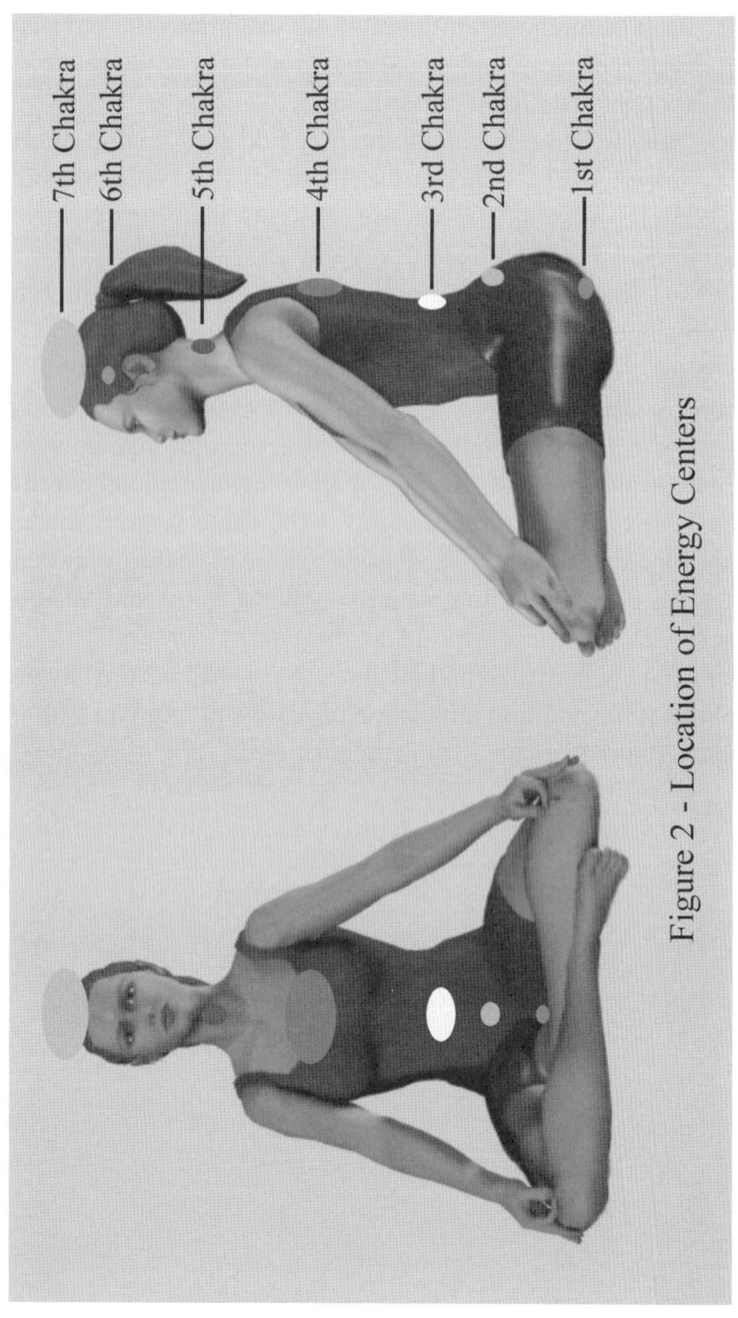

Figure 2 - Location of Energy Centers

The Foundation *Chakra* Model for selfHealing

It has been pointed out in ancient yogic texts, that yogis are those who truly know the *Chakras* or Energy Centers. This exemplifies how critical and potentially complex this whole topic can become. For our purposes, which is the Healing of our physical disEASE, energetic imbalances, emotional bombs and negative mental modifications, only those aspects of the model which are relevant will be presented. There are no discussions about the number of lotus petals in each center, the associated "deities", the magical *mantras* or key derivative sounds, or the many other correspondences which have found their way into texts to satisfy the thirst of the curious. It is not because they are not useful, but only because they are best learned through a reliable teacher, and not through books. As an example, the key sounds or mantras need to be pronounced correctly to have the right effect, and also, an energy transmission needs to accompany the imparting of the sound to provide the impetus towards the desired effect. The only Sound we will be working with in our model is the Sound of *OM*, which is the Universal Mantra given to all of humanity for our evolution.

These Energy Centers cannot be found by dissecting the physical body, but only through achieving higher states of consciousness. Figure 2 gives the location of the *chakras* in relation to the physical body. They are called wheels because of the circular movement of the energies that whirl in and out of them. For our visualization, they are balls of light, and you will be able to feel their circular movement as you progress in the exercises.

These Energy Centers are affected by changes in our internal states, as well as by external vibrations, such as thoughts, words, or actions of others. In the average person, these centers are functioning sub-optimally, and are not harmonized with each other. As the health of the person is decreased through pollution and tension, the more out of tune these centers become. Set 1 of the selfHealing exercises is a means of harmonizing these imbalanced Energy Centers.

Center 1: This is also called the Root Center, and is located at the base of the spine in the perineum and is the root and support of all the other centers. It is connected with the subtle element "earth" representing solidity, and therefore is closely related to the physical body.

Center 2: This is located two inches above the 1st Center along the spine, and is associated with the subtle element water, representing fluidity and movement. This is the center for the emotional body.

Center 3: This is located at the level of the navel, and is associated with the subtle element fire, representing transformation of energy. This center is closely related to the energy body.

Center 4: This is located at the spine at the heart level and is associated with the subtle element air, representing the mind and is the center of the mental body.

Center 5: This is located at the throat and is associated with the subtle element ether, representing consciousness. This is the center for the causal or spiritual body, and is considered the seat of the soul.

Center 6: This is located in the center of the head at the level just above the eyes, traditionally called the "third eye" and is the center for superconsciousness.

Center 7: This is located at the crown of the head and is associated with the Absolute or Transcendent Reality.

The set of Seven *Chakra* selfHealing exercises offered work with the first six centers, and as they become tuned and balanced, they will become more closely linked with the Divine Reality of the 7th Center.

Spiritual Evolution

Each of us is a potential star! More than that, each of us is potentially Divine, and can hold galaxies in the palm of our hands. Such are the teachings of the Ancients. We've been brought up to reject such wild concepts. Wealth and position in society are now the desired goals to strive towards. In our hearts we feel the hollowness of realizing such lofty aspirations, but nonetheless, follow the prescribed rut.

Reality as perceived by the sages is much more glorious. The earth itself is but star-dust, born from stellar debris, and is constantly evolving. From the earth we obtain our bodies, and from our star, the Sun, we receive our life, our soul.

There is an impetus in earth matter to evolve. The physical aspects of evolution have now assumed the loftiness of Darwinian Gospel. Few dispute the evolution from single cell toward multi-cell organisms, from invertebrate to vertebrate, from reptiles to mammals. Although the real story is much more complex for scientific comfort and man's role as yet clouded by yawning gaps, it is a helpful analogy to the immensity that is spiritual evolution. The ancient masters of yoga have always recognized and taught evolution. In fact, the goal of these ancient spiritual scientists was to accelerate the evolutionary process.

Figure 3 shows the state of a "normal human" being limited to body and superficial mental consciousness, and yet controlled by the vaster unknown depths of sub- and un-consciousnesses.

Figure 4 shows how the "individual" body/mental consciousness is only one mode of a vaster framework of evolution to soul consciousness, universal consciousness and finally to naked and empty Being, from which all beings arise.

When human evolution advances to the highest level, the subconscious mind is cleared, ego is dissolved and superconsciousness is awakened. Even more than ordinary human consciousness is light-years beyond animal consciousness, so superconsciousness is beyond the ordinary human intellect, logic and reasoning. Figure 5 shows the relationship of spiritual evolution and physical evolution.

When the highest level of evolution is not only isolated among a few exceptional individuals, but is prevalent in a society, then that society exists completely in harmony with Nature, beyond technology, religion and violence. The energy centers are also related to the corresponding centers of consciousness, as shown by Figure 6, and the self-healing modalities for the *chakras* will have a positive evolutionary effect on consciousness, as well.

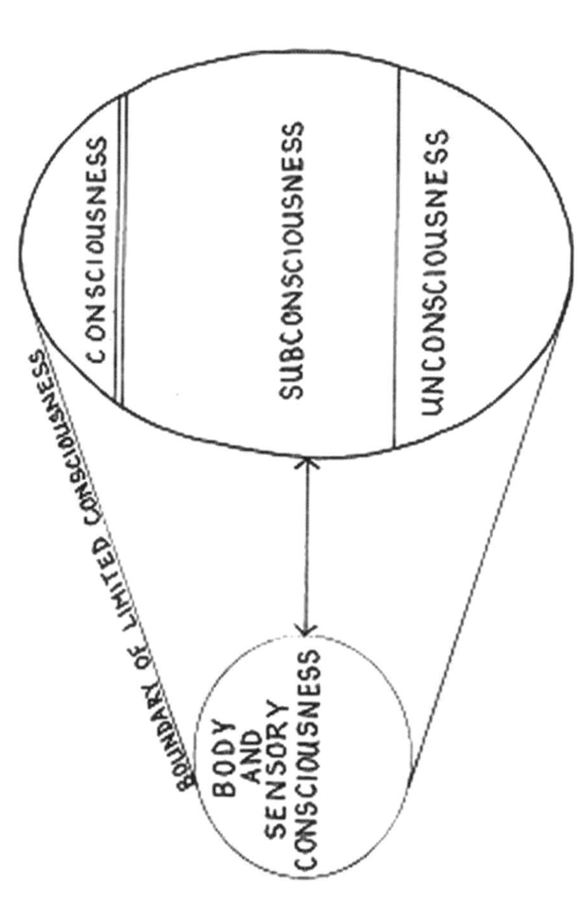

Figure 3 Limited Consciousness

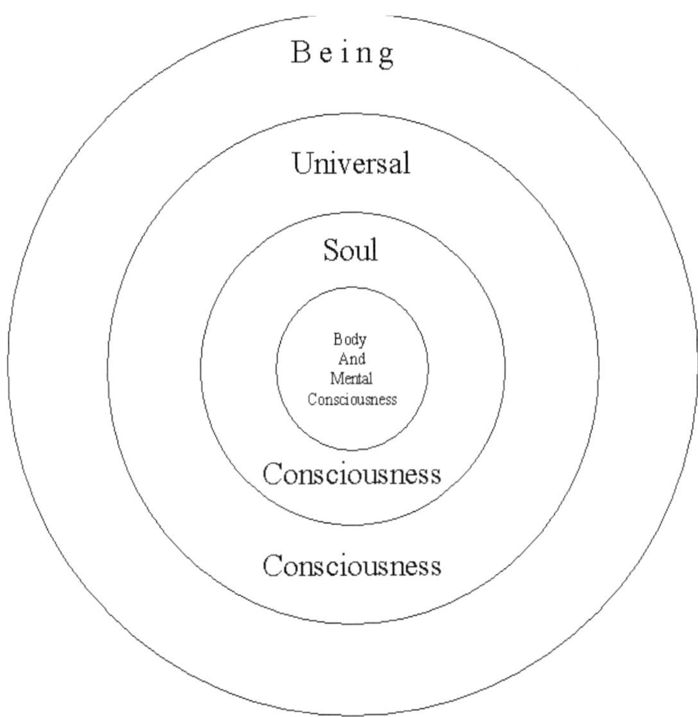

Figure 4 Evolution of Consciousness

Chakra and Consciousness

In the evolution of consciousness there is a corresponding activation and opening of the pranic energy centers called chakras.

From the first base chakra (muladhara) to the navel chakra (manipura) spans the domain of animal consciousness. The so-called unconscious mind of instincts reside in the first chakra while the subconscious mind of impressions and past-life programming or samskaras reside more in the 2nd and 3rd chakras. From this one can realize how deep and strongly embedded are the instincts for survival and reproduction within our chakra system. From the instinct of survival arise the fight or flight response which is accompanied by the fear complex of feelings and emotions, while from the reproduction instinct has arisen the feelings of lust and emotions of desire.

In the 3rd chakra, we see the first glimmerings of individuality, but still from a subconscious level with focus on the instinct of hunger becoming a thirst for accumulation of possessions - from the instinct of survival we seek to control our environment with a roof over our head and a supply of food stored away. From the instinct of reproduction we now seek to control our mate (s) and satisfy our pleasure sensations whenever we wish. The manipura chakra can is the abode of greed.

Of course, you may wonder that I've talked about the negatives of these three chakras without giving any of their positives, for surely they have their counterpoints to balance them.

In actuality, the first two chakras have no negatives – they are natural and animalistic – the negative feelings and emotions come from the impact of our evolved individuality on these first two chakras. In a way, it is our developing human consciousness that has perverted the unconscious and subconscious.

The 4th chakra is the heart chakra or anahata wherein our conscious mind resides – this is the meeting point between the lower animal consciousness and the higher divine consciousness. Here are all the good and bad, for here is where we differentiate ourselves from others and take animal instincts into excess and even perversions – here is where we turn simple hunger into excessive indulgence and obesity and simple sex into rape and pornography. Paradoxically, this is also where our mind can turn towards our True Self, towards the Divine and achieve Divine Love and Compassion, and liberate ourselves into super-consciousness and beyond.

The fifth chakra or Vishuddhi is where super-consciousness resides. This is no longer the mind as we know it, which is limited by three dimensional space and time…limited by the domain of the five senses. Here we can experience higher dimensions of reality unconstrained by thc physical body and senses. This is where we begin to communicate with our True Self. It is still in the realm of duality with object subject distinctions, but at its higher stages the two merge as we approach the realm of the 6th chakra or ajna.

The knowledge and practice of chakra therapy is indeed marvelous, for they contain our suffering in the form of karmic blocks as well as our salvation in the promise of evolution towards higher consciousness as we unravel their mysteries.

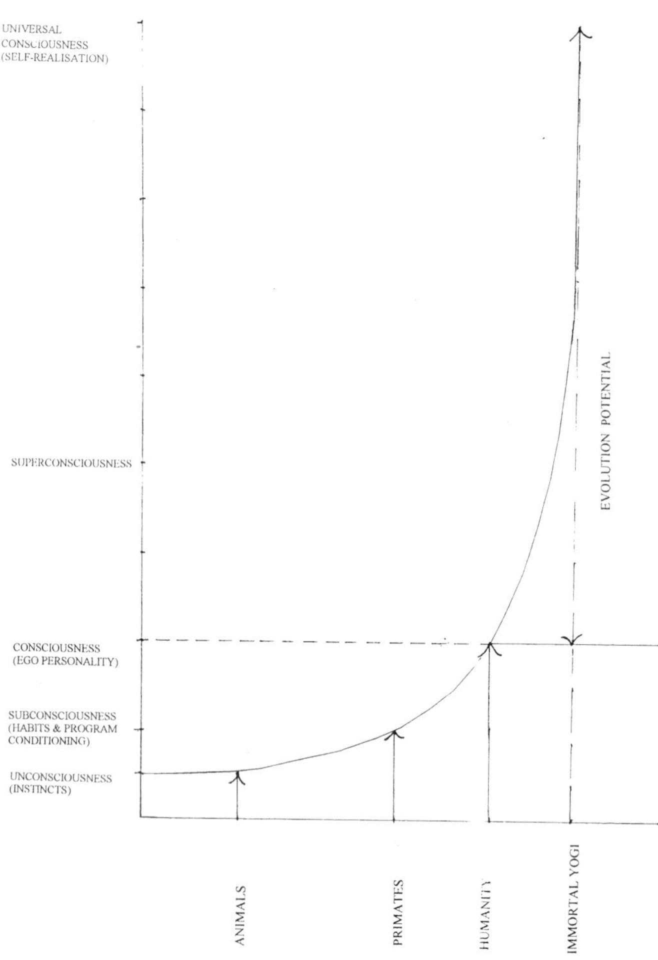

Figure 5 Relationship of Spiritual Evolution and Physical Evolution

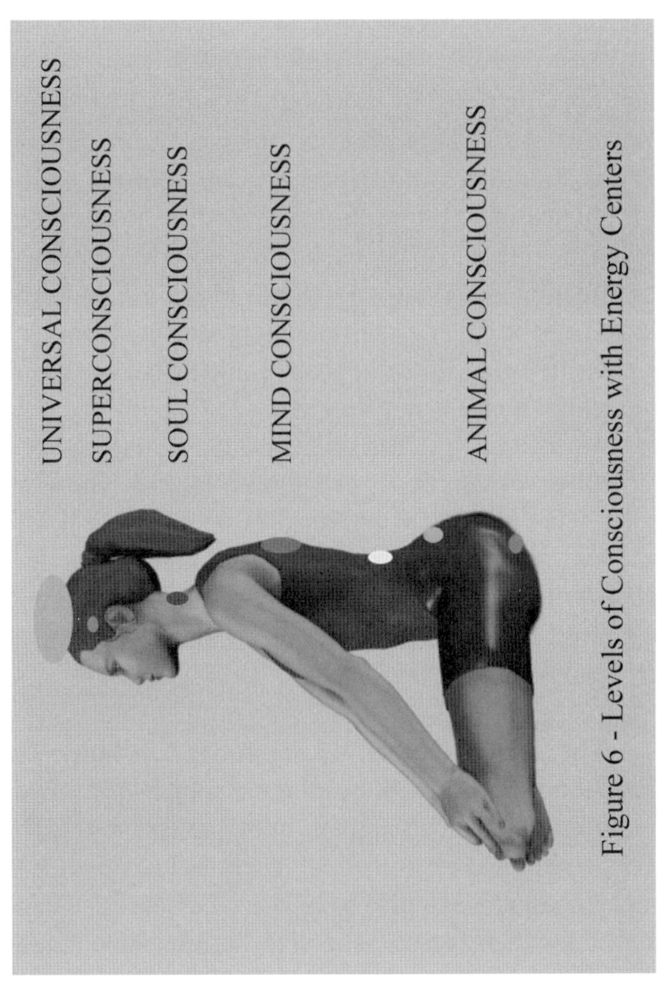

Figure 6 - Levels of Consciousness with Energy Centers

Healing and Health

The exercises given can only be effective if certain precautions are taken to minimize the disruptions to the *chakras* during the self-healing process.

The relationship between the physical organs and the *chakras* works both ways. If the organs are strained or damaged, then the *chakras* become sub-optimal, and vice-versa. By healing the appropriate *chakra*, a slightly diseased organ can be returned to health, but this would be useless if the cause affecting the organ is not removed as well. Sometimes the cause can be a habit, such as indulgence in alcohol which affects the liver. Healing the liver would be a waste of effort, if the alcohol abuse is not stopped.

Diseases can occur at multiple levels. Those at the physical level are mostly manifested due to a weak life-force caused by the impact of stress, over- or under-eating, lack of exercise or lapse in self-control. In general, too much food intake drags down the functioning not only of the physical organs, but of the *chakras* as well.

There are diseases whose roots can be traced to emotional traumas caused by external sources, as well as by negative emotions such as fear, anger, greed, jealousy and hatred, occurring as a result of our reactions to external events. Mental imbalance can also give rise to diseases. Negative mental states such as restlessness, disharmony and ignorance can give rise to both mental and physical distresses.

Past life Karma or the accumulated effects from our past actions can take advantage of temporary physical, emotional or mental turbulence to manifest diseases. The ability to achieve balance through the Chakra selfHealing exercises will help to mitigate the seriousness of these effects.

It is highly recommended that you should cultivate the following habits of good health:

1. Eat more food that provides positive qualities. Food is not just inert dead matter that give up chemicals and physical nutrients for our metabolic needs. All food has innate life-force energy, which will also be assimilated, and can have as strong an impact on your energy systems, as the physical portions of the food. Fruits and vegetables provide higher vibrational energies, which can contribute to the expansion of consciousness. In contrast, the lower vibrations associated with animal-based foods especially those involving violent deaths can contribute negative emotions such as fear and pain into the eater's body-emotion-mind complex, and lead to contraction of consciousness. You should also experiment with some of the food systems that have been verified over many generations such as the Macrobiotic or *Ayurvedic* systems.
2. Eat a balanced diet consisting of not more than 30% each of proteins, carbohydrates, and dairy products [for those who are lactate intolerant, soymilk is a suitable substitute]. Avoid fatty foods, but do use olive oil or sesame oil in moderation. Drink plenty of water to wash away the toxins that tend to accumulate in the body.
3. Supplement your basic diet with vitamins and minerals. This is now needed because of the deficiencies with processed foods and with the paucity in the over-used soil.
4. Minimize the intake of alcohol which stifle reason and

increases desires by reducing self-control and damages organs of the body, such as the liver.

5. Avoid eating late at night. Sleeping with a full stomach will result in undigested food accumulating with the consequent release of harmful toxins, which will overload the body's waste disposal systems.
6. Avoid habit-forming drugs, which weakens the will as well as impairing the harmony of the body-emotion-mind complex. In fact, avoid all allopathic drugs if possible, unless necessary for urgent sicknesses.
7. Sleep regularly and sufficiently. This is the time the body-emotion-mind complex needs to process the physical, emotional and mental poisons that have accumulated during the day. However, too much sleep is to be avoided as it promotes laziness and an inability to deal with life's challenges.

Recommendations for the selfHealing practice

Put aside a set time for the self-healing exercises, either early in the morning before going to work, and in the evening before going to sleep.

Set aside a place for the healing meditation. This can be a small corner of your bedroom which you arrange with a mat and some cushions and a vase with flowers, or can be a separate room.

A number of the healing exercises need to be done with an upright spine, and firm but comfortable sitting posture. It is counterproductive to do healing exercises which involve discomfort.

Sitting pose:

Sit on the floor. Use a mat or rug to ensure a soft sitting area. Fold legs loosely, one in front of the other. Keep the head, neck and spine straight, hands together, with left palm on top of the right palm.

There are seven exercises in this foundation set, with one new one being introduced every week. They generally build on the one from the previous week, and it is recommended that you continue to do the previous ones, as you explore the new one for the week.

A proposed schedule of practice is provided for your reference. Your actual practice will be bounded by the available time you can devote to your own healing and spiritual development.
Table 1

Exercise Week	Set 1A	Set 1B	Set 1C	Set 1D	Set 1E	Set 1F	Set 1G	Set 1A-G
1	10 min	–	–	–	–	–	–	–
2	5 min	10 min	–	–	–	–	–	–
3	5 min	5 min	10 min	–	–	–	–	–
4	5 min	5 min	5 min	15 min	–	–	–	–
5	–	–	5 min	10 min	15 min	–	–	–
6	–	–	5 min	10 min	5 min	10 min	–	–
7	–	–	–	10 min	5 min	5 min	10 min	–
8 onward	–	–	–	–	–	–	–	15-30 min

Empowerment

Traditionally, it is generally necessary to be empowered by an authorized teacher before a seeker can properly, effectively, and safely undertake a prescribed course of practice, which flows from a lineage.

The purpose of the empowerment is threefold:

- **authorize** the practice and gives an initial power boost to the seeker
- **bless** the practitioner and provides help from the positive seen and unseen forces
- **protect** the practitioner from all hindering forces

Babaji, the great Master of spiritual evolution has compassionately given his blessings to this self-healing series and authorizes the seeker to be self-empowered. The effectiveness of your self-empowerment will also be proportional to the degree of your earnestness and to the grace of your own True Self.

Process:

- choose a quiet time, preferably in the morning or early evening
- take a shower and wear clean clothing
- clear a space on a table or an altar
- place a picture of your chosen divine aspect or role-model or even a picture of yourself
- light a candle and softly repeat the following invocation

Invocation for selfHealing Empowerment

I, [your name], hereby invoke the blessings and protection of my Higher Self to remove all obstacles from my self-healing practice.
May my practice be for my highest benefit.
May my practice be for the highest benefit of earth peace.
May my practice heal my physical, energetic, emotional, mental and spiritual bodies.
Om Shanti
Amen Peace

PART 2

7-Step Chakra selfHealing Practice

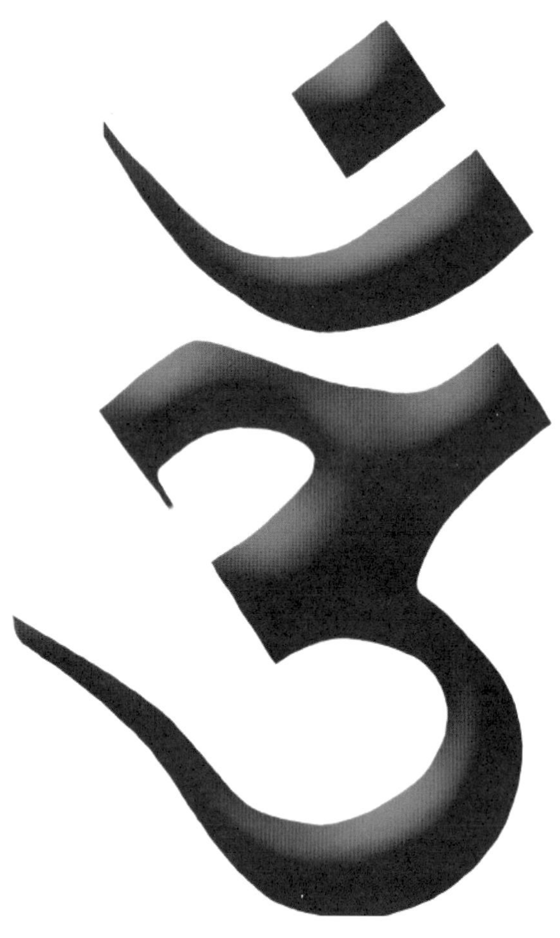

Figure 7

1st Step
Chakra self Tuning 1A
Using the Power of OM

Syllable OM
Symbol of Manifest Divine
Also Divinity Unmanifest
Of Conditioned and Unconditioned
The finite and the infinite
Whoever experiences OM
To non-duality will attain

Prasnopanisad 5.2

OM *Pranava*

Since time immemorial, the ancient sages have transmitted OM as the closest approximation to the creative matrix.

It is called the "unstruck" sound because it is not produced by any mechanical means and is not propelled through space, but is the fundamental **Om**nipresent vibration, called the "music of the spheres" by the Pythagorians. It is the Amen of the Christians.

When properly charged with life-force, sound is the most powerful principle that can bring about all manifestations. Sound is the first manifestation of the Absolute. The Divine Will to create caused a vibration, which eventually became the primordial Sound, and that Sound is OM, from which the rest of the Universe manifested. OM is the basis for all creation, and should it one day cease to Sound, the Universe will be re-absorbed back into the Divine.

Similarly, from the principle that, "As the macrocosm, so the microcosm", our bodies and mind all have the Sound of OM as the foundation. In order to reach our True Self, we need to re-discover the healing Sound of OM within ourselves. The Sound of OM naturally forms the basis of the seven *chakras* or Energy Centers in our individual manifestation. Each *chakra* is able to work with a different harmonic of OM, with the 1st Center sounding at the lowest harmonic, while the 7th Center sounds at the highest harmonic.

To understand the power of Sound, we only have to see how music, which is one of its physical manifestations, affects animals, and how human beings are soothed or agitated by music. Scientific experiments with beds of sand have shown a particular sound will form a definite and specific shape, and different sounds form different shapes.

OM is the manifest representation of Divinity and the Universe of Creation. It is the primal sound from which the universe evolved. The chanting of OM quickly relaxes the mind and body, generating spiritual power and accelerating evolutionary transformation.

The sound of OM is composed of the combination of the vowel sounds of *A* and *U*, with the letter *M*, and the sound of silence. Innumerable correspondences have been created by the ancients for the four parts of OM : *A* represents the physical world and wakeful state, *U* represents the Astral world and dream state, *M* the causal world and deep sleep state, while the silence represents the spiritual world.

The form of OM is shown in Fig. 7, consisting of three curves, one semicircle and a dot. The bottom curve denotes the wakeful state, the upper curve the deep sleep, and the curve in between signifies the dream state. The dot represents the Absolute state of Super-consciousness while the surrounding semicircle represents the conditional world of conventional reality.

The complete syllable OM is considered by the sages to be the highest knowable reality, and those who know it are said to attain all their desires – it is the source of everything and nothing. The ancients have said that by uttering OM as one departs the body at death, liberation from the cycle of rebirth will be attained.

It is because of the power and effect of OM that it is used as the basis for all of the Self-healing exercises in this set, to activate and "tune" the energy centers.

Repeating OM
The one creative syllable
Thinking of me
Divinity Manifest
Departing the body
The way of Truth he goes

Bhagavad Gita 8.10

Posture

Unless otherwise instructed in the exercises themselves, the posture recommended is one of comfortable and stable sitting.

The physical discipline of sitting correctly is itself of great benefit for the energy system, as well as enhancing mental discipline and improving the powers of concentration.

There are four postures that can be used, as shown in figures 8 and 9:

1. The least difficult and strenuous in the beginning is sitting on a chair. Make sure the chair's back is straight, but sit on the front edge of the seating area, with your back straight without resting it. Let your legs rest comfortably over the edge of the chair, with the soles of your feet balanced flat on the floor.
2. Easy pose or cross-legged posture is the customary relaxed sitting posture on the floor. You may wish to sit on a cushion so as to elevate your pelvis above your legs to decrease the pressure on the legs.
3. Perfect pose is the yogic meditation posture that is highly recommended. Sit with your legs stretched forward. Bend your left leg and place the heel of the left foot against the perineum.

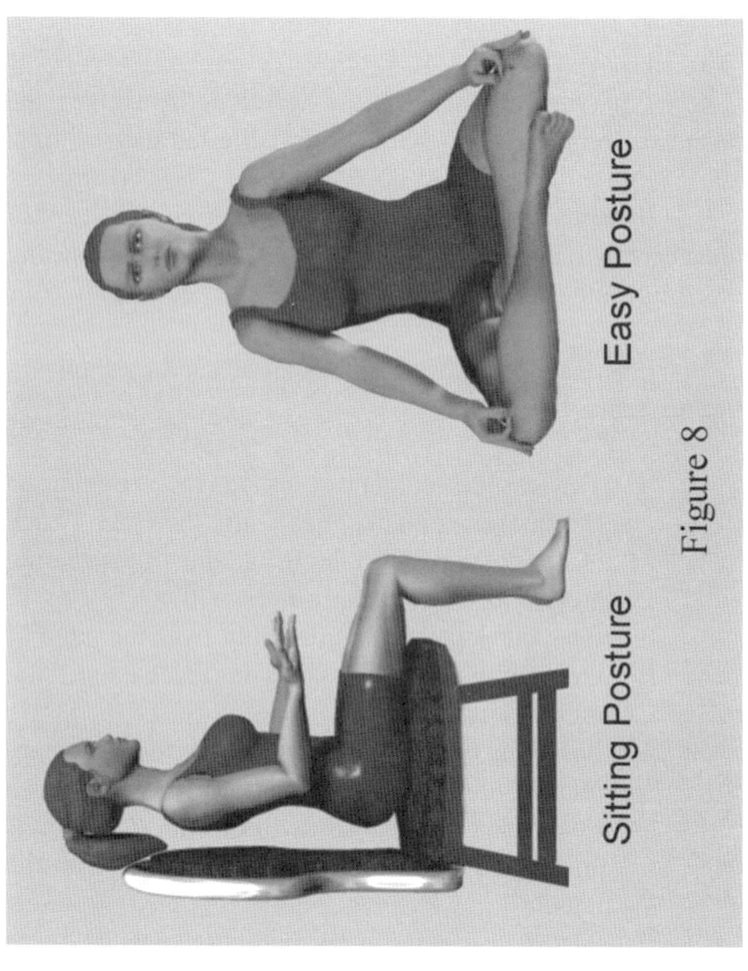

Figure 8

Bend your right leg over the left and place it on the left thigh with the right heel resting against the genitals. The knees should be touching the floor.

4. The lotus posture has great benefits, if you can get into it without too much strain. Extend both legs forward and bend your right leg carefully over the left, placing it on the left thigh, as close to the groin as possible. Bend your left leg at the knee and place the left foot on the right thigh. It will take some practice to be able to get into and stay in this posture comfortably. A modified and simpler posture is called the half-lotus, where the left leg is simply tucked in under the right.

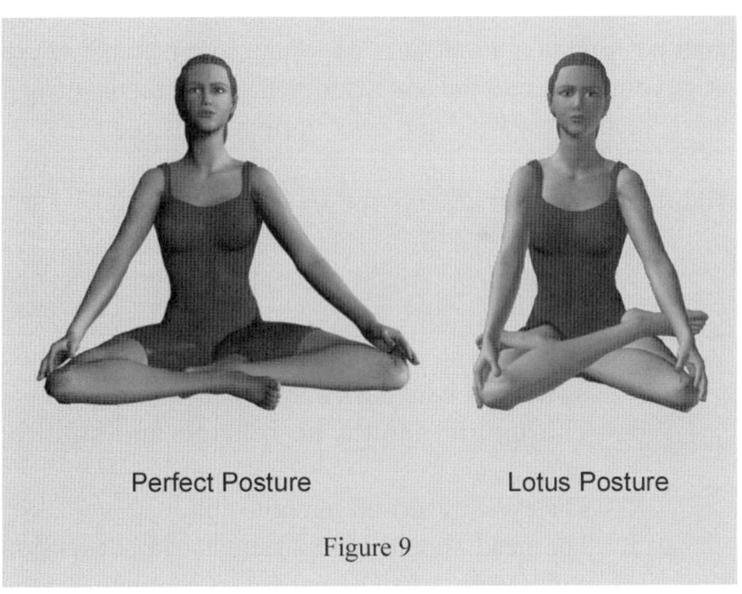

Figure 9

Another consideration during the practice is the position of the hands and arms. There are three simple positions that can be used with any of the four postures, as shown in Figure 10:

1. Open receptive: Rest your hands on your knees with the palms facing up.
2. Place the back of your right hand on top of your left palm with the thumbs lightly touching each other.
3. Interlace your fingers together and rest them on your lap.

Whichever variation and combination of posture and hand position you adopt, it is important to remember not to press your arms into the body, and relax your shoulders and chest, keeping the head and neck upright and steady.

Additional points to observe for good posture:

1. The back is straight without undue strain, so that energy can flow freely.
2. The shoulders are relaxed and not hunched forward or bent backwards.
3. The mouth should be relaxed and slightly smiling.
4. The eyes are closed but relaxed.
5. The head should be held erect without tension with the neck tucked in ever so gently.

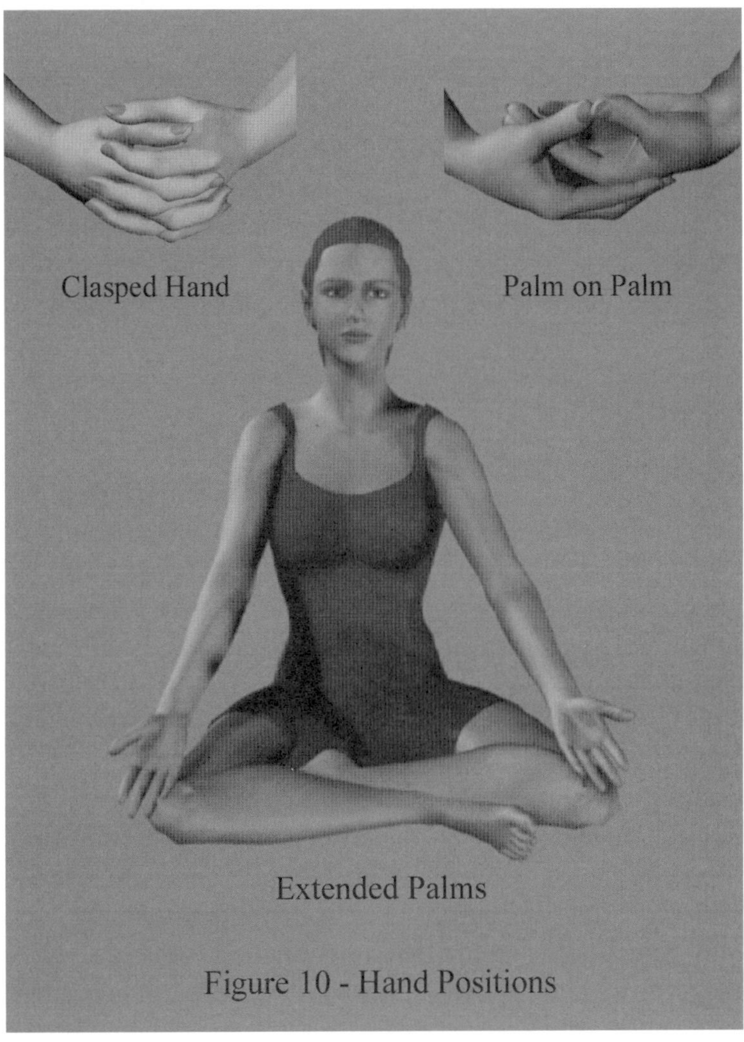

Figure 10 - Hand Positions

Chakra self-Tuning [Set 1A] Technique

Preparation:

Sit in a comfortable posture with back straight and eyes closed. Focus attention on each *chakra* position along the spine. In the beginning it might be useful to touch the location and get a physical sense of the position. Touch the base of the spine where the tailbone ends with the fingers of your left hand. Move up 2 inches and rub where the 2nd chakra would be, and so on.

Attention and feeling are key ingredients for this experiment. The key catalytic ingredient is the sound of OM. Repeat this sound aloud a number of times until you are comfortable with it. You can find out more about this **OM**nipresent source of all matter and energy in the next section.

Procedure:

Focus your attention on the Root or 1st *Chakra* position. Mentally repeat OM twelve times. This can easily be done with three sets of four OMs each. It is important to hitch your mind to this repetition without letting it wander. After the twelve OMs, allow yourself to feel the vibration at the 1st *Chakra* for a few seconds to a minute, depending on the time you have for the total tuning procedure. Remember to be relaxed and not tense you body.

Move your attention to the 2nd *Chakra* and after establishing your focus there, repeat mentally twelve OMs. Allow yourself to feel the vibration at this new point. If you don't feel anything, don't get discouraged, as you will be more sensitive while you continue your practice over the week.

Now move to the 3rd or Naval *Chakra,* on the spine, just opposite from the navel, and repeat the twelve OMs with attention and feeling.

Don't stay at any center for too long, as you may start to have experiences and feelings which you should put aside at this stage, and move to the next center.

The 4th *Chakra* is at the heart level along the spine. You should be able to feel the vibration of the heart itself at this *chakra*, not to be confused with the vibration of the *chakra* or of OM itself. Move to the Throat Center after completing the twelve OMs at the Heart *Chakra*, and feel the twelve OMs at this location. The upward movement continues to the sixth *chakra* or Third-Eye Center. At this center, after repeating the twelve ascending OMs, retain your attention here for 1 minute, and then repeat twelve more OMs – the descending OMs, as you reverse your course back down the *chakras*. You will resound the twelve OMs at the throat, heart, naval, 2nd and 1st *Chakras*. At the end of the cycle, you will have performed 144 OMs, seventy-two up and seventy-two down.

Now raise your hand above your head, taking a deep breath, vocally intone OM.

Rest peacefully and feel the OM all around you, for as long as you feel comfortable.

Effect:

OM is the cosmic hum of the Universe. In this exercise, the *chakras* are tuned to this creative hum, returning them to a healthy and higher state of vibration. By tuning the energy centers to OM, they are activated spiritually, which in turn will heal the mental, emotional, energetic and physical bodies.

2nd Step
Chakra Balancing 1B
Using the Power of Healing Hands

I have come here to give you rest
I have come here to keep you safe
With my hands I bring you strength
With my hands I drive away your disease
They encompass all healing energy
As the tongue precedes speech
My gentle, encompassing, healing hands
Makes you whole

Arthavaveda Book 4, mantra 13

Healing Hands

From pre-historic past down to the present, the "laying of hands" has been an instinctive as well as superconscious response to "healing" at various levels. Instinctively we put our hands to where we have pain or are hurt. Somehow we believe that this will help. Those who have been privileged to receive spiritual initiations or empowerments know that often the climax of such ceremonies is the touch of the Master's hands. What is the significance of this rather multifunction appendage?

From the physical perspective, the palm and fingers of each hand has a large number of nerve endings and are consequently extremely sensitive. A blind person reading Braille is an inspiring sight.

From the perspective of energetics, it is a scientific fact that energy is strongest when concentrated at point or at long sharp shapes such as the apex of a triangle, and can be transmitted from point to point as is demonstrated by the lightning discharges of a static electricity dynamo.

You can easily verify the energy potential of your hands by rubbing your two hands together for a minute and then sitting receptively with eyes closed, place the two hands palm facing, about three inches apart. Feel the connection between the two palms, moving them slowly closer without touching, and then with awareness separating them further. Do this several times. You should be able to discern the energy field around the hands.

If you can accept that we are all Beings of Energy, we should be able to transmit or redirect healing energy to different parts of our body or to the body of others. Our hands are the natural tools for doing this.

What is the source of the healing energy being transmitted?

During the energy balancing exercise, the hands are redistributing the energy from the different *chakras*. When you are trying to heal another person, the wise healer will act as an energy conduit for Universal Healing Energy rather than try to transmit his or her own life-force energy.

Chakra Balancing [Set 1B] Technique

Preparation:

Create your self-healing space by sitting quietly for a minute and then performing *Chakra* Tuning [Set 1A] for 5 minutes. Then place a clean sheet on the floor and lie down with a light pillow under the head.

Procedure:

1. Balancing the Navel and Heart Centers:
   Lie down on your back. Place your left hand on your navel and your right hand on your chest. Relax and keep your eyes closed and your attention on the hands and the two centers. Keep your fingers together rather than spread apart, but without tension in the hands. Feel the gentle vibration of these two centers through the palm of your hands for three minutes. Then focus on the navel below your left palm. After about ten seconds, move your attention to the back opposite to the navel where the 3rd energy center is located. Then move your attention up the spine to the 4th or heart center and finally to the front where the right palm is resting on the chest. Return to the navel and complete this energy circuit four more times.

2. Balancing the Sacral and Throat Centers:
   Continue lying down. Move your left hand down to the pubic area and move the right hand up over the throat. Be careful not to put too much pressure on the throat.

Feel the synchronization of these two energy centers for three minutes. Then focus on the left pubic area where the left palm is resting. After about ten seconds, move your attention to the back where the sacral center is located and rest there for about 10 seconds before moving up the spine to the throat center. Finally, move forward to the front below your right palm. Return to the pubic area and complete this energy circuit four more times.

3. Balancing the Forehead [Third-eye] Center:
   Sit up slowly. Keep your back erect. Place the left palm over the back of the head covering the medulla oblongata, and the right hand over the front of the forehead. Focus on the vibration as it brings the two poles into mutual balance. You will also be able to sense the Root *Chakra* at the sacrum, as it is closely connected with the back of the head.

4. Balancing the Root or 1st Center:
   Assume the normal sitting posture. Stretch out your hands in front at the chest level, with palms facing up. Fold the hands at the elbow and gently place the palms on the shoulders. Feel the vibration at the perineum and feel the harmony with all the other energy centers for five minutes.

Effect:

Our energy centers or *Chakras* are normally balanced relatively to each other. With stress, tension, emotional reactions and other negative stimuli, they become imbalanced and operate sub-optimally. Set 1B corrects the imbalance.

3rd Step
Chakra Color Tuning 1C
Using the Power of Color

One who perceives a disk of light
Like a jewel at the navel
Is a knower of Yoga
Flashes with a golden light
Like Lightning

Yoga Chudamani Upanisad 9

Light and Color for Healing

There has been a renewed interest in recent years in the effect that color or the lack of a particular color plays in our physical and emotional health. Ancient cultures have always understood the need to be surrounded by the appropriate color vibration.

In India, the wearing of colored gemstones to cure health problems or to ward off karmic calamities has been accepted by the general population for thousands of years. Chinese Fung Shui or the Science of Harmony with the Surrounding Energy System has provided for the right colors to be used in the different directions to best effectuate harmony for the desired results in health, and other fields of human concern, such as wealth.

Different cultures have settled on different colored clothing for certain occasions – western tradition uses white, the color of purity for weddings and black for funerals, whereas the purity of white is the color used in Chinese funerals and red, the color of energy and life is used for Chinese weddings!

Color is the visible vibrations of light energy. All light emanates from the sun, the great ocean of light and the source of all life. The Seven Rays are of the visible spectrum: red, orange, yellow, green, blue, indigo and violet. Not only the physical world but also the energetic, emotional, mental and spiritual planes are sustained by the Sun's White Light.

From an individual's point of view, this means that color affects us physically, energetically, emotionally, mentally, and spiritually. Our thoughts and feelings vibrate to color and to the fields around our five bodies, which some label the auras, are continuously throwing out all manners of colors.

Why does one person prefer certain colors and are repelled by others? All matter radiates light and has a color vibration, which is continuously emitted and has an affect based on the reaction from the "color consciousness" of the person.

The "color consciousness" is the aggregate of the "color state" of the energy centers or chakras. This "color state" is a complex of the balance and health of the energy centers.

To illustrate how complex it can be, take for example someone who is very spiritually inclined, who gravitates towards blues and violets, but may be deficient in the reds and orange of life and vitality. He may follow a conscious plan to surround himself with reds and orange to increase his physical health, or he may follow his subconscious inclination to avoid the life and energy colors. There are many variations to how a person will react to an excess or lack of particular colors in their life.

There are some healers who believe that diseases are primarily caused by the malfunction of the color balance within the sick individual. Treatment would then consist of identifying the missing color(s) and using various means to achieve balance, such as wearing the appropriately colored clothing and gems, or re-furnishing the home or office to inject the needed colors. Depending on the seriousness of the condition, over a period of time, the body, mind and soul will be revitalized with the defects and infirmities healed.

The first energy center is associated with the Red. This is the color of life, and is a positive vibration, which acts as a healing agent for diseases of the blood and circulation. It will also act to dispel mental depression. Red is a spectrum of vibrations composing a band of frequencies. It can arouse the primary instincts and primal desires in the subconscious mind, and this can have negative impact on a person's behavior. On the other hand, it can stimulate energy, strength and physical power and inspire courage and enthusiasm. Action is the characteristic of life, and Red is the color of action.

Orange influences the 2nd energy center and is connected with the spleen. It functions as an agent for absorbing and distributing vital energy, and corrects digestive problems. It is an antidote for repression and limitations, promoting self-confidence and positive thinking.

The 3rd energy center is keyed to yellow. The color yellow works on the nervous system, and on the liver. It promotes creativity and can correct skin and nerve problems.

Green is the color of balance and is primary at the heart center. It influences blood-pressure and heart action, and stimulates kindness and peace.

Blue is the color of consciousness and is primary at the 5th energy center of the throat. It promotes truth and peace of mind, and corrects fevers and headaches, as well as certain types of inflammation because of its soothing effects.

The 6th center at the third eye is associated with indigo and violet. Indigo is associated with the pineal gland, and is influential with the organs of sight, hearing and smell. It is the color of the soul, and it an antidote to fear, as well as correcting diseases of the eye, ear and nose. Violet is the color associated with the pituitary gland and is the color of superconsciousness, as well as physically correcting cerebral and neurological problems.

From the above brief summary, you can have an appreciation for the impact that color has on our life. However, it is necessary to be cautious in their use, or over-reliance on their effectiveness, because our human holistic system is very complex, and color is only one part of it.

Refer to Figure 11 for *Chakra* Colours.

Visualization

Every one of us has the ability to visualize, but not all of us have utilized this ability consciously.

Very simply, visualization is of two types:

1. Using our memory to recall the image of an object that we have seen before.
2. Using the imagination to construct an image that we have not seen before.

Whether we are aware of it or not, whenever we visualize something, whether it be a recent vacation moment or a childhood memory, there is an emotional reaction which occurs simultaneously.

Therefore we can use visualization to help arouse certain states of mind that can affect our energy centers and the five bodies, to bring about healing.

In the following set of exercises, it is necessary to be able to visualize balls of different colors at the energy centers. If you experience difficulty in visualization, you might want to practice by drawing a circle and coloring it in green. Look at the green ball, and then close your eyes. Try to imagine the green ball and hold the image for a few minutes. Good imagination and visualization skills are very important in many meditations techniques, and it will be worthwhile to acquire facility in their use.

Chakra Color Tuning [Set 1C] Technique

Preparation:

Perform *Chakra* Tuning and Chakra Balancing for 5 minutes each. Sit up after finishing the Balancing set to continue.

Procedure:

1. Visualize a rosy red ball of energy at the Root *Chakra*. Hold this image and mentally repeat twelve OMs.

2. Visualize a snow-white ball of energy at the third eye center. Hold this image and mentally repeat twelve OMs.

3. Visualize an orange ball of energy at the 2nd *Chakra*. Hold this image and mentally repeat twelve OMs.

4. Visualize a deep blue ball of energy at the throat center. Hold this image and mentally repeat twelve OMs.

5. Visualize a golden ball of energy at the navel center. Hold this image and mentally repeat twelve OMs.

6. Visualize a bright grassy green ball of energy at the Heart Center. Hold this image and mentally repeat twelve OMs.

7. Continue to hold the image of the green ball of light at the heart center. Let the ball of light expand so that your whole body is immersed in this healing green orb. Feel the vibration of OMMMM all around you for one minute. Let the green orb of light dissolve into your heart.

Effect:

Each *chakra* has a distinctive characteristic color related to its rate of vibration. The blue color of the throat *chakra* is at a higher vibration than the red color of the root *chakra*. By visualizing the color associated with the energy center, it is quickly returned to its optimal state of health. This exercise is particularly effective after a day at the office with its attendant stress and strain.

4th Step
Chakra Rejuvenation 1D

Using the Power of Postures

Like rubbing two sticks together
To make fire
Use the body as the lower fuel-stick
OM syllable as the upper fuel-stick
Strike them against each other
The fire of self-realization arises

Svetasvatara Upanisad 1.14

The Healing and Spiritual effects of Physical Postures

Physical postures are not only essential for toning the muscles, tendons and joints of the body, but also help to regulate the harmful effects of stress and maintain balance in meeting life's challenges. They massage the internal organs and glands to stabilize the physical body. A regular practice of a yogically planned set of postures such as that of Babaji's Kriya Hatha Yoga can help eliminate poor health.

The postures selected in Set 1D are specifically associated with the Energy Centers, and are not intended to cover all parts of the body or replace a full-set of posture practice.

Certain precautions should be followed when practicing any of the postures:

1. Do the postures in stages to avoid straining the muscles by going too quickly into the final stage.
2. If any particular part of the posture is too difficult at this time, less stretching is indicated until there is increased flexibility.
3. Breathe naturally. Never hold the breath. Frequent holding of the breath will weaken the heart, by reducing the flow of oxygenated blood to it.
4. Relax after each posture for as much time as the posture is held. This is an essential part of the

posture. This is what differentiates a healing posture from calisthenics.

5. Focus on the physical body, its sensations and tensions. Relax the muscles not needed to hold a particular posture in place. Do the postures slowly and deliberately, as a witness. Remain continually aware of the body and its reactions. Do not allow the mind to wander to other subjects.
6. Practice before meals and never with a full stomach.

The practice of the postures with continuous awareness introduces you to meditation.

Chakra Rejuvenation with postures [Set 1D] Technique

Preparation:

Perform 5 minutes each of the previous three sets of exercises, and then stand up to stretch your hands and walk in place for 1 minute to warm up the body. Place a comfortable mat on the floor before proceeding.

Procedure:

1. Forehead or third-eye center: Salutation
   Refer Figure 12
   Sit on heels with arms at sides. Lean forward, touching the forehead to the floor. Stretch arms back towards feet, palms upward. Breathe naturally and focus on the 3rd eye center, repeating OM twelve times. Feel the vibration through the contact of the forehead on the floor, and relax in this position for a few moments before gently raising your head and getting up into a standing position. Relax in the standing position and continue to feel the third eye center.

2. Throat center: Shoulder Stand
   Refer Figure 13
   Lie flat on the back, arms parallel to the body. Raise legs so that they make a right angle with the body. You may wish to stay in this position if your have difficulty going to the next stage. Then using your arms to support your

lower back, raise body straight up on shoulders so that it makes a right angle with the head. Chin is pressed tightly to hollow of throat. Breathe naturally and focus on the throat center, repeating OM twelve times. Feel the vibration and pulsing at the throat. Hold this posture for about three minutes. Gently relax down, and lie flat for 30 seconds. If this posture is strenuous for you, try to do it against the wall, and using the wall to support the legs.

3. Heart center: Reverse Posture Mudra [topsy-turvy posture]
   Refer Figure 14
   Lie on the back, arms at sides. Slowly raise legs until they make a right angle with the body. Keeping elbows on the floor, raise torso and support hips with hands. Legs are vertical. Pressure is at heart level and not at throat. Breathe naturally and focus on the heart center, repeating OM twelve times slowly. Feel the vibration of the heart energy center. If the posture is strenuous, you can do rest your legs against a wall to support you. Hold the posture for about three minutes.

4. Navel center: Camel Pose
   Refer Figure 15
   Sit on the heels, knees slightly apart. Reach back and grab heels with hands. Push buttocks and abdomen forward, arching back and bending head back slowly. If this posture is too difficult, try leaning back and placing both hand on the buttocks to support yourself, instead of reaching for the heels. Focus your attention on the navel energy center, and breathing naturally, repeat OM twelve times. Feel the vibration at the navel center, and hold this position for about 3 minutes.

5. 2nd *Chakra*: Locust Pose
   Refer Figure 16
   Lie face down on your front, keeping both legs together and your hands by your side. Raise both legs together from the hips, using the your hands to balance. Focus your attention on your 2nd energy center and repeat OM twelve times there, feeling the vibration, even after you've finished. Hold the posture for as long as you can. Relax your legs down slowly and rest for about three minutes, releasing all stress, and continuing to feel the energy center. If it is difficult for you to hold both legs up, an alternative is to raise the left leg up, lower it, and then raise the right leg up, in a scissors movement for about seven times. With both legs on the floor, focus on the 2nd Chakra and continue practice of OM in the relaxed position.

6. 1st *Chakra*: Balancing coccyx poise
   Refer Figure 17
   Lie down on your back. Raise your legs off the floor, but keep your seat still touching the ground. Clasp both hands together under the knees, and sit up, balancing on you seat with your forehead close to the knees and the feet pointing forward and slightly up. Continue to balance on your buttocks. Focus you attention on the tailbone and perineum, repeating OM twelve times there. Continue to feel the vibration, and hold the position for 3 minutes. Relax back down on your back, lower arms and then legs to the floor.

After the completion of the whole set, continue to a relaxation pose, in order to release any stress that may have been introduced by the exercise, since your muscles may be unused to these positions.

From the 6th posture, lying on your back, turn your head slowly from side to side a few times.
Relax your neck and head by stopping the movement.
Grip the thumb of your right hand with the fingers, forming a fist, and squeeze your whole arm, then relax.
Raise your right forearm a few inches off the floor, keeping the elbows down, and let it down.
Raise the whole right arm off the floor, keeping the shoulders on the floor, and let it down. Do the same movements on the left side.
Then move the toes of your right foot back and forth, and then spreading them apart. Do the same with the left foot.
Rotate the feet together and outwards using the hips — both feet will be rolling on the heels.
Raise the right leg as a whole off the floor, a few inches, and then let it fall. Repeat with the left leg.
Relax in this position for a few minutes, feeling your body, energy centers, and any emotions.
Breathe into any stress and release all physical, energetic, emotional and mental blockages.

Effect:

Combining the physical movement and postures with the *chakra* visualization and healing vibration of OM is the most effective method to re-integrate the physical body with its life-force centers. Through this re-integration, the physical body enjoys a regenerative healing.

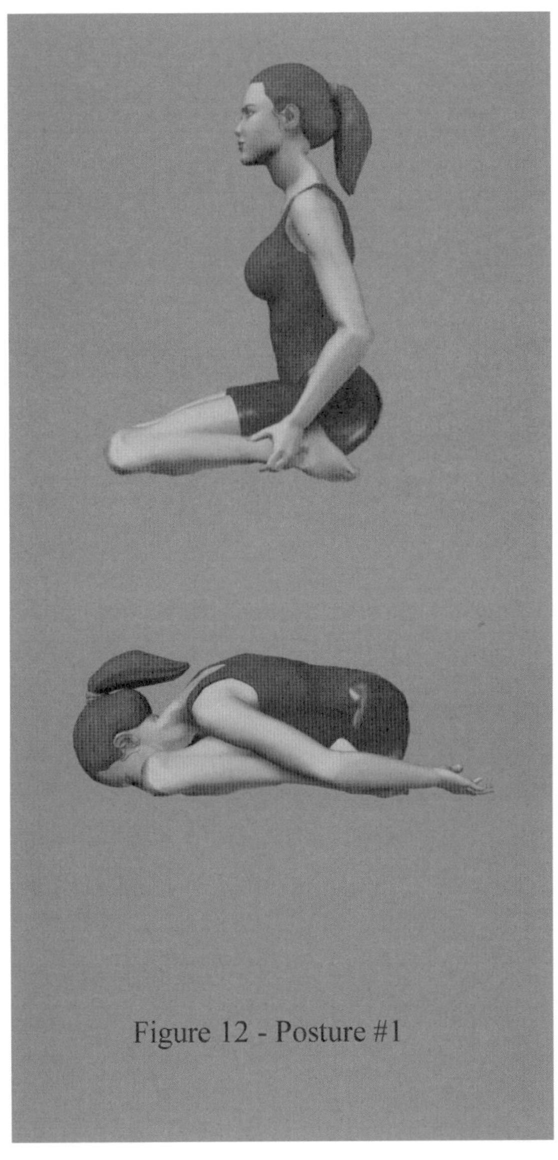

Figure 12 - Posture #1

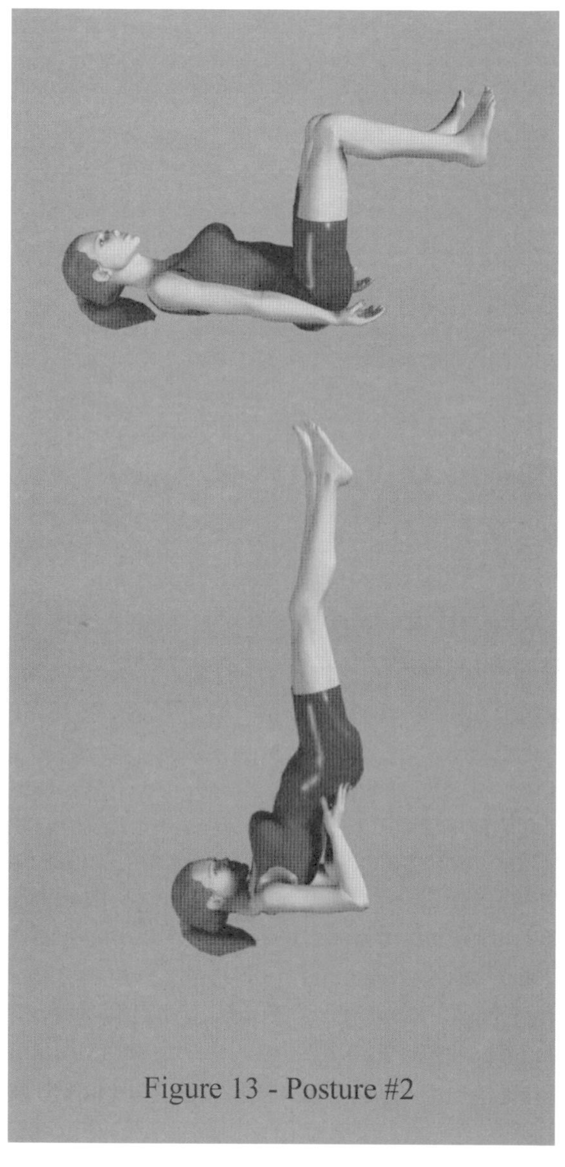

Figure 13 - Posture #2

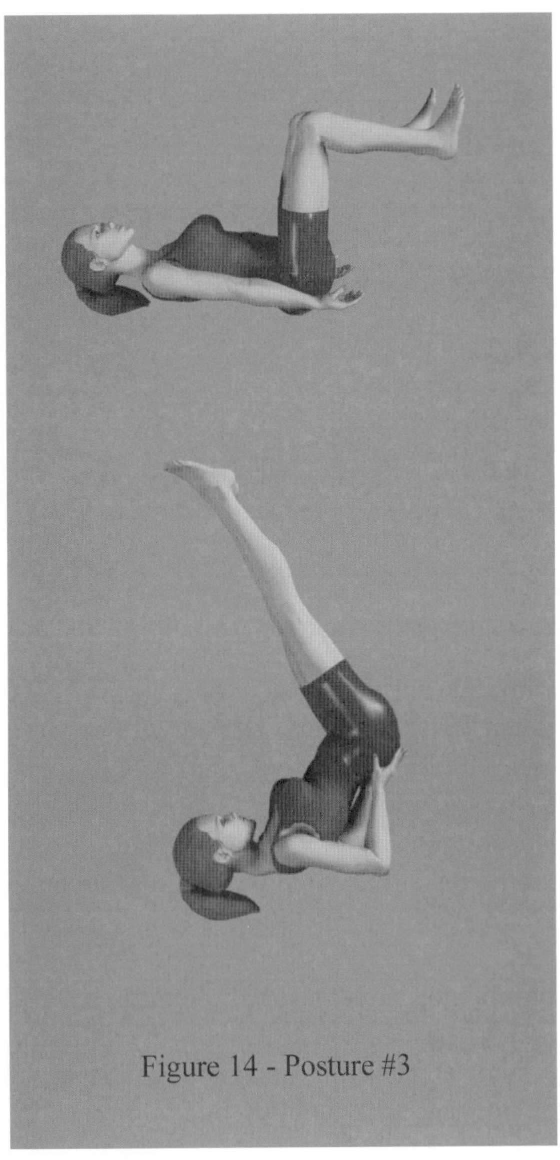

Figure 14 - Posture #3

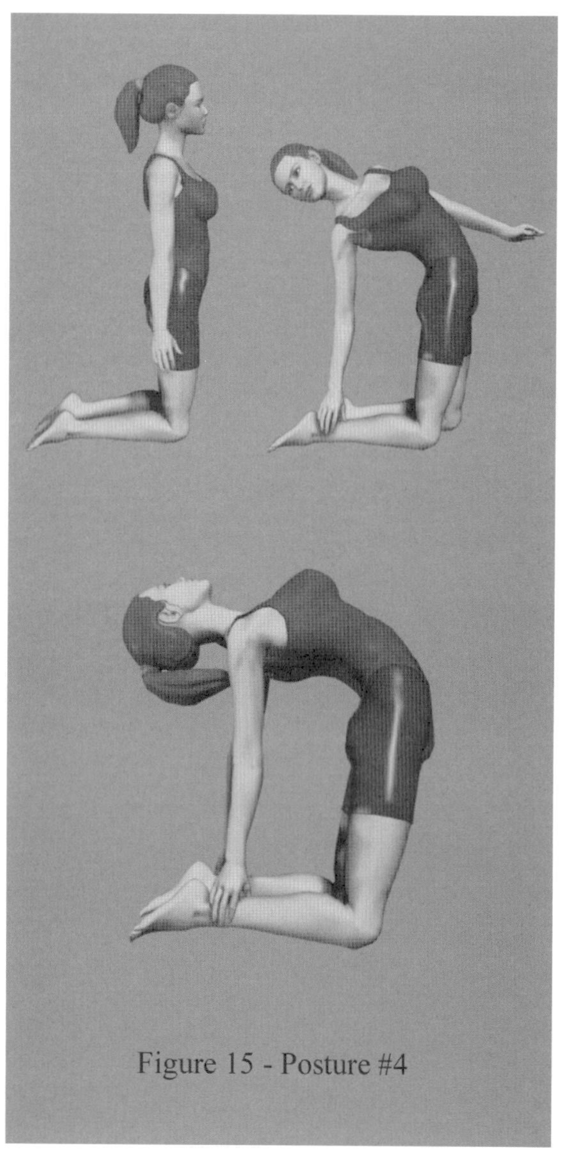

Figure 15 - Posture #4

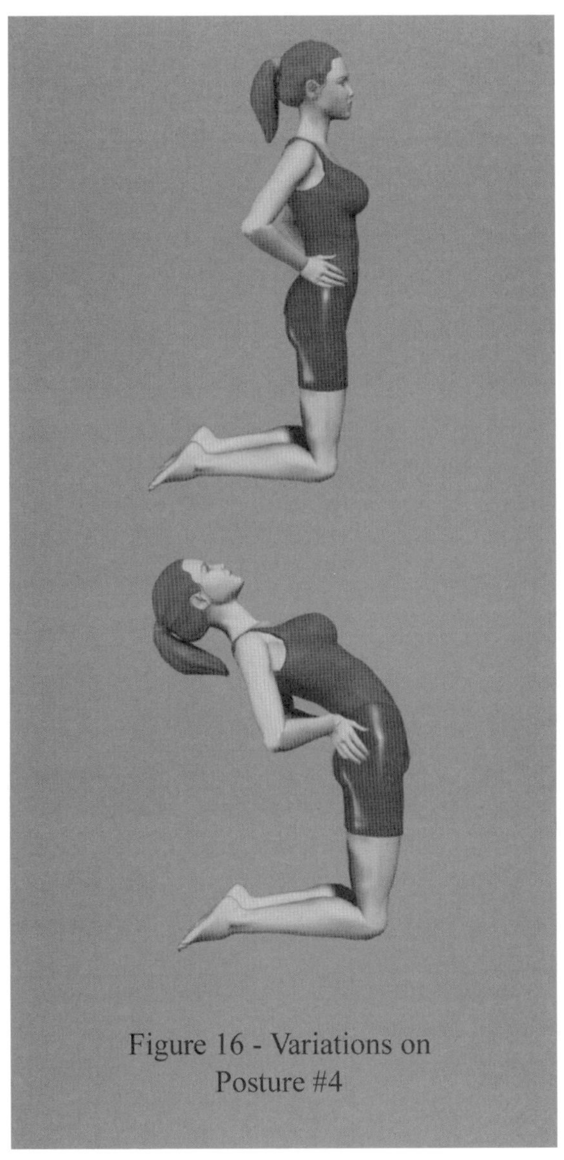

Figure 16 - Variations on Posture #4

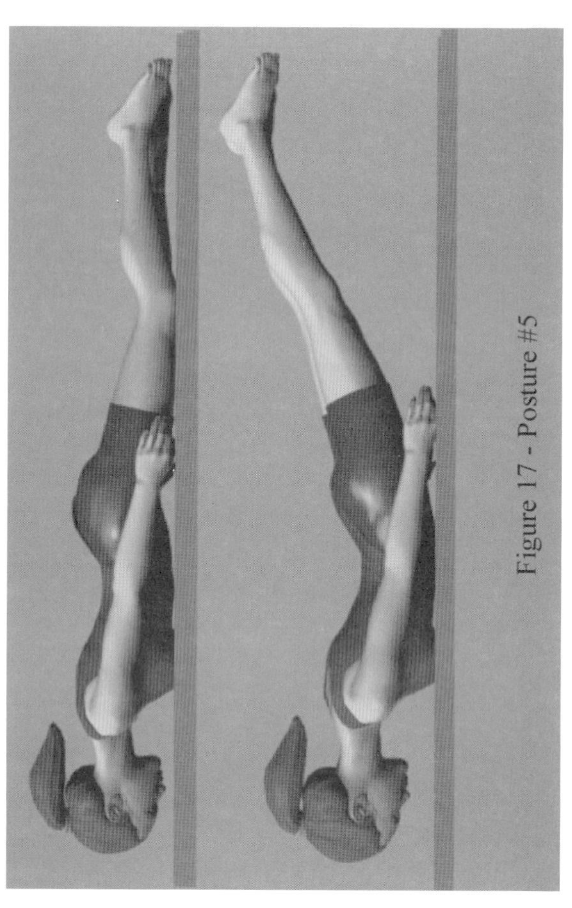

Figure 17 - Posture #5

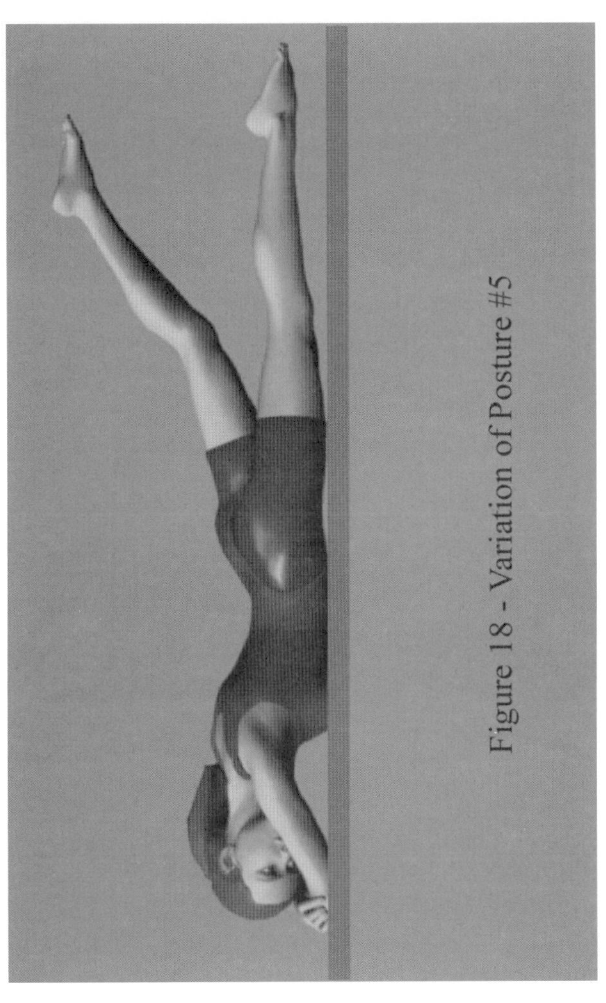

Figure 18 - Variation of Posture #5

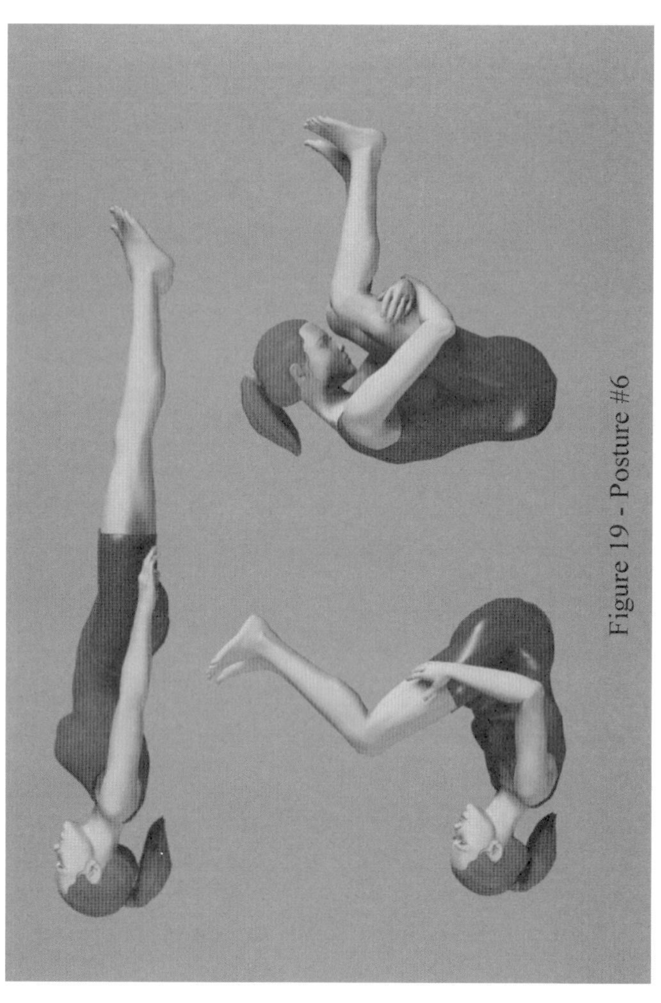

Figure 19 - Posture #6

5th Step
Chakra Emotional Detoxification 1E
Using the Power of Positivity

Speak the truth
Follow the path of righteousness
Do your duty now
In married life, look after your children
Integrate spiritual and worldly realities
Never stop learning, share with others
Be grateful to the Divine
Praise those who've come before you

Taittiriya Upanisad

Achieving Emotional Balance

Emotional Healing is an important aspect in the growth of consciousness. There is a tendency in spiritual paths to sweep "under the rug" or ignore emotional issues, with the consequence that even after years of endeavor, spiritual aspirants can still be caught up in unpleasant emotional states.

The expansion of awareness requires the integration and channeling of emotional life towards the experience of more positive effects. Negative and unhappy emotions such as anger, jealousy, fear, depression and guilt are left behind. Instead the energy which gives rise to these states is experienced in a more refined and purified form as joy, peace, love and compassion. There is a stream of manifestation for all emotions and the cultivation of awareness of this stream of arising is the beginning of emotional control.

In order to exercise emotional control, it is necessary to understand the way that emotions arise. If we can observe the arising of an emotion, we will see that it was caused by a desire, which in turn was caused by an instinctual urge. Humanity shares the same primary instinctual urges, which are the need for food, self-preservation, sex and sleep. These are the drivers for our need to nourish the body, avoiding bodily hurt and defending its well-being, the creation of new life for the preservation of the species, and revitalization of the body.

Unlike animals, which just express their urges in a straightforward manner, "the pinnacle of evolution on earth" has misused his imagination to create an unending number of objects, situations and experiences to try to indirectly satisfy these urges. We have created all sorts of conditions and criteria for food – the look, taste, texture and smell. The desire for status, power and accumulation of possessions are all manifestations of the basic urge for self-preservation.

Emotional pleasure arises from the satisfaction of a desire, and an emotional dependency results from the habitual connection of pleasure with the satisfaction. Unpleasant emotions or displeasure result from the experience of situations or objects, which we would like to avoid, leading to a habitual aversion for those situations or objects. All of us have things we like and those, which we dislike, and it is not always clear how it all came about that we react within the set program.

Anger arises when a particular desire is unfulfilled, and if this frustration continues, unreasoning violence in thought, word or deed, rears its ugly head. Under the constraints of modern society, anger is suppressed, leading to stress, a leading cause of ill health such as high-blood pressure or mental illnesses. There are those schools of thought that promote the release of "negative emotions", supposing that such cathartic exercises would release stress and promote a positive effect. Aside from leaving a person drained for a certain period, and therefore incapable of further emotional outbursts for that period, no long-term benefit seems to occur. The positive experience seems to indicate that it is the channeling of the emotional power, which is valuable, has long-term effects, and should be pursued.

Jealousy and envy arises when our desires are fulfilled by others. We begin to long for or covet the experiences or possessions of those who seem to "have it all". Such a reaction arises when we feel an emptiness within ourselves, caused by our inability to connect with our Center, the Divine within us, the True Self. There is no desperate grasping for external validation when one feels the inner completion, the joy of Self-realization.

Fear arises from the instinct for self-preservation – the fight or flight instinct, which in modern society generally translates to a flight reaction of some sort.

There are countless fears, and most of us spend our whole life reacting and moving from one to another. Ironically, the very fears themselves can cause that which is feared to occur. Fearing attack from others, can lead to behavior, which invites the attack. Fearing rejection from others can lead to a negative way of approaching relationships, bringing on the rejection feared, and so on, in a vicious cycle of catch 22. The only solution is to eliminate the fear, which in turn will eliminate the danger and the rejection. Obviously, this is easier said then done, as the causes of our fears are very deep, and are the very basic addictions and dependencies, which arise from our imagination and externalization of internal issues which we have refused to face or change. Clinging to phenomena and fearing change leads to suffering and pain. Freedom from fear arises when in higher consciousness, we can experience the "still center of the universal no-mind".

There are many other emotions, such as greed, pride and depression, and we need not to delve into them at this time. What is of more concern, is the methods of channeling emotions. Spiritual devotion is one method for channeling emotional energy through chanting, prayers and study of holy texts. Another method is the use of Insight or Intellectual discrimination, so as to see through the emotions, and experience the Still Center, thereby achieving integration and freedom.

The way of developing positive emotions as an antidote for negative emotions is very helpful in the beginning stages of self-healing. These positive emotions are centered around the primal urge for completeness, for Self-realization, the desire for higher consciousness, for truth. These positive emotions can be developed to the extent that they can swallow up all the other desires, and the consequent negative emotional reactions.

Chakra Emotional Detoxification [Set 1E] Technique

Preparation:

At a minimum, perform the 3rd set for 5 minutes and the 4th set for 15 minutes. Then assume the sitting posture of your choice and with eyes closed and focused inwards to proceed.

Procedure:

1. Root *Chakra*: The negative emotion that needs to be detoxified from this energy center is fear, and the positive antidote is courage.
   Repeat the following affirmation 3 times loudly, 3 times softly, and 3 time mentally, while focusing on the 1st *Chakra*:

   OM
   I am fearless
   I meet life's challenges with Courage

2. 2nd *Chakra*: The negative emotion to be detoxified from this energy center is lust, and the positive antidote is harmony.
   Repeat the following affirmation three times loudly, three times softly, and three times mentally, while focusing on the 2nd *Chakra*:

   OM
   I am complete

Free from Dis-Ease
Harmony in Duality

3. 3rd *Chakra*: The negative emotion to be detoxified from this energy center is greed, and the positive antidote is abundance.
   Repeat the following affirmation 3 times loudly, 3 times softly and 3 times mentally, while focusing on the 3rd *Chakra*:

   OM
   I need nothing
   I am filled with life's abundance

4. 4th *Chakra*: The negative emotion is hatred, and the positive antidote is love.
   Repeat the following affirmation 3 times loudly, 3 times softly and 3 times mentally, while focusing on the 4th *Chakra*:

   OM
   I am empty of hatred
   I love X and X loves me [here X is your current bitterest "enemy"]
   The Divine loves me.

5. 5th *Chakra*: The negative emotion is anger, and the positive antidote is compassion. Repeat the following affirmation 3 times loudly, 3 times softly and 3 times mentally, while focusing on the 5th *Chakra*:

   OM
   I am joy
   Joy is Divine
   May all Beings be happy and filled with joy
   May all Beings be free from Suffering

6. 6th *Chakra*: The negative emotion to be detoxified from this center is pride, and the positive antidote is sacrifice. Repeat the following affirmation three times loudly, three times softly and three times mentally, while focusing on the 3rd eye center:

   OM
   I forgive all those who have harmed me
   I forgive myself who has harmed others
   The fruits of my action, I offer to the Divine

Effect:

Cleanses the accumulation of negative emotions and habit patterns.

6th Step
Chakra Energization 1F
Using the Power of *Prana*

All life is under the control of *Prana*
The cosmos is sustained by *Prana*
Protect us like a mother
Give us prosperity and wisdom

Prasnopanisad 2.13

Freedom from Life-Draining Forces

There are two sources of energy for the body: indirectly from food and directly from life force. It can take hours to convert food into energy, but the your Will can immediately generate the necessary energy from the Universal Energy reservoir. In order for you to tap into the reservoir, not only must you understand the nature of the relationship between the body life force and the universal creative matrix, but you must also be able to feel and experience it.

The Universal Energy that permeates the galaxies and our world, is the same energy which is unceasingly vibrating in our five bodies. This life force energy is called *Prana*. In its cosmic aspect, it is also called *Shakti*, and in its microcosmic aspect, where it represents the individual's highest potential, lying dormant in the 1st energy center, it is called *Kundalini*. The active aspect of the *Kundalini-Shakti* which enlivens the body is a 10-fold *Prana* driving the primary physiological functions of the body. There is *Prana* in our bodies, and there is *Prana* outside our bodies. We are swimming in a sea of *Prana*, which can be absorbed through our breath and through our skin.

As you've been practicing the self-healing exercises so far, there will be a marked increase in your energy level and awareness. However, in order to sustain and maintain this higher state of well-being, it is necessary for you to drop or avoid situations and habits which can decrease your energy level and put you back into a lower state, in which you might be more susceptible to disease. In addition to avoiding life-draining situations, one should cultivate life force enhancing habits and situations.

What are the life force draining habits and situations which should be avoided? What to cultivate?

1. Avoid places which have a lot of negative energy. Our system can get depleted trying to resist and fight off the negativity. Bars, brothels and casinos are examples of places where lust, greed, anger and fear permeate palpably. There are very few places in our modern society where you can find positive energy – try going to different churches, and find one where you feel good after spending some time there.
2. The pollution in our cities deprive us of life-giving *prana*. Try to spend time in the fresh air of parks and mountains. The amount of *prana* is directly proportional to the oxygen in the air.
3. Avoid the company of people who have bad habits because they have low energy levels, and will drain you of your higher energy, much like a "vampire". All of us have had the experience of being drained after spending time with someone. This does not mean that we do not bring comfort to those in need, which is a conscious effort to help others. Cultivate the companionship of those who have abundance of positive energy, and who can help you in your path to self-healing. This seems obvious, but it is surprising how often the committed seeker will avoid the company of other seekers for no discernable reason, other than prior habit patterns. They will continue

old relationships which have ceased to have any meaning because of divergent interests, out of respect for old behavior.

4. Avoid idle chatter and loose talk. The spoken word is full of energy. There are great masters of yoga who recognizing this had achieved self-realization, in part, by keeping silence for extended periods of time, to build up their energy level. Sometimes, we feel so excited that we are drawn to share with someone, and feel drained afterwards. It is always best to cultivate a middle path of non-excess.
5. Avoid over indulgence in sensual pleasures. Eating too much is bad for your health, just as drinking too much, or having too much indiscriminate sex. All these sensual activities will drain you of your Prana. Cultivate a moderate appetite in all things.

All of us have different needs. Each of you must bear the responsibility to implement the kind of healthy life force enhancing plan that appeals to you.

Chakra Energization [Set 1F] Technique

Preparation:

Perform *Chakra* Balancing and *Chakra* Color Tuning for 5 minutes each

Procedure:

1. Visualize a Golden Ball of energy at the 3rd or Navel center. Feel the vibration of this ball of light and mentally repeat twelve OMs.
2. Expand the golden ball so that it surrounds your whole body.
3. Keep awareness of the golden ball and repeat 12 OMs at the 3rd Eye center, then 12 OMs at the Throat center, 12 OMs at the Heart Center, 12 OMs at the Navel center, 12 OMs at the 2nd center, and 12 OMs at the 1st center.
4. Dissolve the golden ball into the Navel center
5. Visualize your whole body as a hollow vessel, and let the golden ball expand to fill the whole body inside. Perform the *Chakra* Tuning with OM at each energy center from the 1st up to the 6th, and then from the 6th down to the 1st center. After 1 round, dissolve the golden back into the Navel center. Relax for a few minutes.

Effect:

Revitalizes the *chakras* with life-force energy.

7th Step
Chakra Transcendence 1G
Using the Power of the Subtle Universal Elements

From the Divine arise Space [gravity]
From Space arise Air [kinetic energy]
From Air arise Fire [radiation]
From Fire arise Water [electricity]
From Water arise Earth [magnetism]

Taittiriya Upanisad 2.1

The Five Subtle Elements and Man

The ancient Masters of Wisdom perceived reality directly, and have transmitted their insights on cosmic evolution through countless generations. They perceived that cosmic consciousness gave rise to Universal Energy which then manifested into the five Universal Elements – Material Building Blocks of Space, Air, fire, Water and Earth - which became the atomic building blocks of all matter and energy, through a process of grossification. It is important to keep in mind that the translation of the these words is imperfect and should not lead you to confuse them with their common usage. When the Masters talk about Space, they are more closely pointing out the universal force of gravitation then anything resembling “open space”.

From Universal Energy, the vibration of OM caused the appearance of Space, which moved and created AIR, and from the function of it’s movement, SPACE created the Fire element. From the heat of Fire, Space dissolved and liquefied and gave birth to water. When the Water element solidified, Earth is formed. The whole of the material Universe is formed by the combinations of these five Elements. It should be noted that these five Elements are not visible particles, but through a process of grossification, became present in all matter and energy. They refer to the etheric, gaseous, radiant, fluid, and solid states of matter and the principles of space movement, light, cohesion, and density.

As an example, the planet Earth is formed with a greater proportion of the gross aspects of the Earth Element.

The five bodies of man are formed by various proportions of those five Elements. In the physical body, the solid structures such as bones, muscles, skin and hair are derived from the Earth Element. From Water Element, all the fluids and secretions are derived, while the Fire Element rules the digestive and metabolic systems. All movement of the body is governed by Air, while cavities are the province of Space.

The Five Elements also manifest in the Five senses, providing for all perception of external environment. Space, Air, Fire, Water, and Earth are related to hearing, touch, vision, taste and smell respectively. Since the human body (all 5 bodies) are a manifestation of the Five Elements, a balance of harmony of these are required for healing and health, as well as for spiritual realization.

The path to Self-realization must start through an understanding and passage through the Primary Elements.

Table 2 shows the Elements and their corresponding senses and organs of action and the relationship with the specific energy centers.

TABLE 2 – FIVE ELEMENTS

Chakra	Element	Sense	Sense Organ	Action Organ	Organs of Action
5th Center	Space	Hearing	Ear	Speech	Organ of Speech
4th Center	Air	Touch	Skin	Holding	Hand
3rd Center	Fire	Seeing	Eyes	Walking	Feet
2nd Center	Water	Taste	Tongue	Procreation	Genitals
Root Center	Earth	Smell	Nose	Excretion	Anus

Among these five subtle elements,
from the principle of inertia,
the five gross elements are produced.

By the principle of Activity,
And from subtle Space, the organ of speech is born
the hand is born form subtle Air,
the leg is born from subtle Fire,
the genitals are formed from subtle Water,
and the anus is formed form subtle Earth.

By the principle of Clarity,
the organ of hearing,
the ear is evolved from subtle Space,
the skin (organ of touch) is evolved from subtle Air,
the organ of sight (eye) is evolved from subtle fire,
the organ of taste (tongue) is evolved
from subtle water,
and the organ of smell (nose) is formed
from subtle Earth.

Chakra Transcendence : Tuning with the Subtle Elements [Set 1G]

Preparation:

Understanding the subtle elements.

Look at the figures of the Elements in the Appendix and practice visualizing them in their appropriate colors.

General Procedure for all the Chakras:

1. Eyes Open
   Look intently for about 3 minutes at geometric representative of the element
   Gaze without blinking as far as possible, but not straining yourself to the point of tears. Repeat the appropriate words for the element aloud seven times.

2. After-image
   Look up from the figure and keeping your eyes open, look at a white surface such as a wall or a white piece of paper. There will be an after image. Look at the after image and repeat the appropriate words for the element until the after-image has disappeared.

3. Eyes Close
   Visualize the image of the element and repeat the words for the Element for about 3 minutes.

On the first day, focus on the Space element, second day on Air, 3rd day on Fire, 4th day on Water, 5th day on Earth element, then on the sixth day, focus on all five Elements starting from Earth to Space. On the 7th day, start from Space back down to Earth, spending about 3 minutes on each element.

Specific Procedure:

1. Throat Center:
   refer figure 24 for blue circle of space element
   Repeat the following words:
   OM
   Space is limitless and boundless

   After completing the three processes outlined above in the general procedure, keep the eyes closed and feel the throat chakra. Visualize the blue circle of the space element in front of you. Feel the image connected with the throat center and visualize it merging with the throat center for about one minute.

2. Heart Center:
   refer figure 23 for green star of air element
   Repeat the following words:
   OM
   Air is freedom and Movement

After completing the three processes outlined above in the general procedure, keep the eyes closed and feel the heart chakra. Visualize the green star of the air element in front of you. Feel the image connected with the heart center and visualize it merging with the heart center for about one minute

3. Navel Center:

   refer figure 22 for red triangle of fire element
   Repeat the following words:
   OM
   Fire is heat and light

   After completing the three processes outlined above in the general procedure, keep the eyes closed and feel the navel chakra. Visualize the red triangle of the fire element in front of you. Feel the image connected with the navel center and visualize it merging with the navel center for about one minute.

4. Sacral Center:

   refer figure 21 for silver crescent of water element
   Repeat the following words:
   OM
   Water flows and holds

   After completing the three processes outlined above in the general procedure, keep the eyes closed and feel the sacral chakra. Visualize the silver crescent of the water element in front of you. Feel the image connected with the sacral center and visualize it merging with the sacral center for about one minute.

5. Root Center:

    refer figure 20 for yellow square of earth element
    Repeat the following words:
    OM
    Earth is firm and fruitful

    After completing the three processes outlined above in the general procedure, keep the eyes closed and feel the root chakra. Visualize the yellow square of the earth element in front of you. Feel the image connected with the root center and visualize it merging with the root center for about one minute.

Effect:

Connect with the principles of solidity, fluidity, light, freedom and boundlessness. Freedom from the limitations of the rigidity, instability, and destructive tendencies.

Part 3

The Next Steps

Once you've successfully utilized the self-healing tools provided in this program, you are ready to expand your experiential base. Follow your intuition and find the path that best helps you accomplish your spiritual goal.

You may want to continue practicing some or all the exercises that you have been doing, or integrate one or more of them into your regular practice. The key is to continue some sort of regular practice, whether it is for 5 minutes or 8 hours, progress can be made through consistency. Enthusiasm rises and ebbs like the tide, and should not be relied on to sustain your practice.

Find a Teacher whom you can rely on to lead you to the Light.

In following section, I've attempted to give brief descriptions of various paths which might be pursued. It is up to each person to find the path that best suits their temperament.

When you've completed the selfHealing program in this workbook, you've taken a measure of control over your own physical, emotional, mental, and spiritual well-being.

Further progress is entirely in your own hands.

You may want to repeat the program several times and deepen your healing. There is much to explore in these timeless self-healing techniques.

There are layers to the *Chakra* healing program which can be explored. Mountains of volumes have been written on the *charkas* or energy centers, and their corresponding colors, elements, *bija mantras*, Sanskrit characters, ruling deities, auxiliary symbols etc. You may refer to various translation and excerpts from the *Sat Chakra Nirupan*, such as "Serpent Power" by Arthur Avalon. However, hardly any effective techniques are given for using these correspondences in a coherent manner, as they are only passed directly from teacher to student. New age writers have resorted to inventing exercises from their own inner experiences and there are a plethora of such, some useful, others not, with the seeker hardly able to sort the pearls from the chaff. It is only through personal instruction that the higher levels of *Chakra* healing can be effectively transmitted. selfHealing workshops exploring the 2nd and 3rd levels of *Chakra* power evolution may be of interest.

Besides utilizing the *Chakras*, there are other power sources of self-healing. Workbooks on selfHealing through self-Discipline, Postural Integration and Solar Power are also available from Alight Publications.

If you are primarily interested at this time in Healing exercises, there are excellent schools of Chi Kung offering a balance and strengthening of the energy systems in the body. Another popular solution are the new age physical posture schools of "Popular Western Yoga", which can provide a strong foundation for good health.

For those drawn to spiritual healing and the paths of transformation, there are a bewildering array of choices. You will be guided by your inner friend, who has been awakened by the program which you've just completed. In the following pages, I've briefly sketched a few of the major paths to help you make an informed choice towards your evolutionary path. Sometimes your choice will be determined by where you are and what or who you are drawn to, and sometimes you will be driven to travel great distances to satisfy your thirst. The only sure thing, is that it will never be dull !

I've confined myself to describing those paths which are streams from the *Sanatana Dharma*, the eternal fountain of life from which all the yogic systems have their roots. Yoga is not tied to any religious system per se, but sometimes inevitably become colored with layers of cultural and religious attitudes, as well as powerful symbols of the areas from which they flourished and developed. However, the mark of a true spiritual path is that the core or essence does not depend on these extraneous layers and can be adapted to different cultures and times without losing their effectiveness.

Into blinding darkness enter those
who only work
Into greater darkness fall who solely meditate
Different fruits from action and meditation
Overcome death by devotion to life in the world
Achieve immortality through meditation
The wise have explained the true path
Practice both self-less action and meditation

Isa Upanisad 9,10,11

The *chakras* are the keys to health and spiritual evolution

There is probably no other yogic tool as important as that of the energy centers or *chakras* since they have important roles for both the physical, emotional and mental health of a person as well as being pivotal in attaining to higher conscious states.

There are hundreds of *chakras* in the energy body but the six major ones along the subtle spine are the most crucial. This is because they are the repositories of our karma. The six *chakras* are the muladhara at the perineum (connected to the base of the spine), swadhisthana at the sacrum (about 3 inches above the base), manipura at the back corresponding to the navel, anahata or heart center, vishuddhi at the base of the neck and ajna in the middle of the brain. There is of course the 7th *chakra* called sahasrara *chakra* or thousand-petalled lotus at the top of the head but this center is that of perfection and does not have any function.

It is very useful to learn the names of the *chakras* themselves as they have mantric significance and the repetition of their names causes vibrations at the energy centers.

Each of the *chakras* is responsible for certain bodily functions – the muladhara is responsible for the physical body as a whole, the swadhisthana for the emotional body, the manipura for the energy body, the anahata for the mental body and the vishuddhi for the causal body.

There is also overlapping of functionalities in that although muladhara has overall control of the physical body, it also has minor functions for emotions, energy, mental states and karmic memory. For instance, this first *chakra* rules the emotions of fear and courage.

It is important to understand that these energy centers are very subtle pranic structures and are maintained directly by the life-force energy. When the life-force energy is depleted, then they cannot function properly and then every aspect of our life that they control will be hurt. On the flip side, when we do, say or even think something negative which resonates with a particular *chakra*, then it becomes depleted of prana! Of course when we apply ourselves positively, then more prana will go to the *chakra* concerned.

In the subtle energy body, the *chakras* are connected together by fine filaments of energy called the nadis. These nadis act like the arteries and nerves in the physical body, and they can be blocked or even damaged so that some parts of the subtle body might not be getting the life-force needed. However, since they are energy filaments, they can be repaired, redirected and even grown by the power of prana – this aspect is essential for healing purposes.

For the spiritual evolution and development of higher consciousness, the main energy channel called sushumna nadi flows along the spine and through the 6 major *chakras* that we have been discussing. It is through this central channel that the latent kundalini shakti has to rise up for the bliss of samadhi and the flowering of super-conscious states. Therefore, each *chakra* has to be sufficiently opened and filled with life-force energy before the kundalini will be attracted up to it. We need to work progressively upward in the normal course of events in order to raise the kundalini but in practical safety terms, it is recommended to try to open the 6th *chakra* or ajna first, in order to provide the positive pull from above.

If the higher *chakras* are shut and we open up the lower ones, then there may be difficulties encountered in the first three *chakras* which may challenge the practitioner's ability to cope. There are practices which work on all 6 *chakras* progressively without over-emphasizing on any one at a time and these are the kind of practice that I recommend. Even when one is putting greater emphasis on one particular *chakra* in order to work out certain problems, it is always a good idea to exercise all the other *chakras* regularly to some extent. For instance, if you are spending half an hour on the heart *chakra*, combine it with a five minute each practice on the other five *chakras*, making up almost an hour.

Working on the *chakras* is a life-long pursuit but one of the most worthwhile that anyone can embark on. The healing affects can occur very quickly but due to our karmic inertia and habit patterns, the energy centers cannot be so easily opened and developed for spiritual purposes. However, it is a necessity for Self-Realization and so persevere in your efforts.

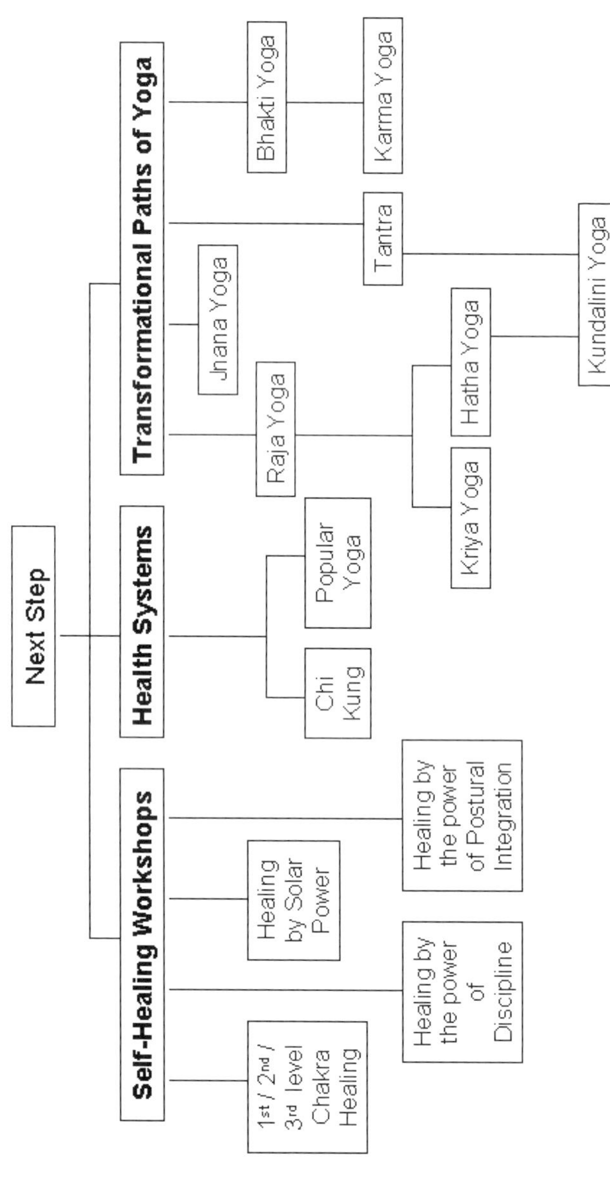

Table 3 Next Step

2nd Level *Chakra* selfHealing Workshop

The healing power of Om is the key ingredient or catalyst in the 1st level. The next phase introduces the specific controlling sound or *Bija Mantra* of each of the seven energy centers.

A mantra is a scientific formula given in a sound or series of sounds which can produce a specific physical energetic, emotional, mental, or even spiritual effect. The spiritual masters have passed these formulas through a personal initiation or empowerment from ancient times. Even though some semblance of these *Bija Mantras* or "Seed Mantras" have been written down in books, it is crucial to successful practice to have them given personally from a teacher with the correct pronunciation and empowerment. Moreover the actual practice using these *Bija Mantras* are not really written down and is handed down to students after they have demonstrated proficiency in the fundamental techniques.

Besides the *Bija mantras*, there are also other *mantric* sounds which can be utilized to bring more power to the *chakras*.

3rd Level *Chakra* selfHealing Workshop

In addition to the controlling *Bija Mantras* or Seed sounds given in the 2nd level, the *Chakras* also have specific energy modes which are symbolized by geometric figures and the forms of universal energies denoted as Gods or Goddesses.

However, the keys to unlocking the Power Potential of the *chakras* are only given to those who are qualified and blessed by good luck to meet someone who can guide the ultimate practice.

This practice leads to the dissolution of all blockages and the awakening to Self-Realization, the Ultimate Healing.

selfHealing through Discipline

It is said by the *Siddhas* or Perfected Yogis that the amount of happiness in One's Life is proportional to the effort at Self-discipline. Most of our suffering, grief and unhappiness are a result of inappropriate actions caused by an undisciplined mind.

In this context, disciplining the mind is not just a matter of willpower or forceful restraint, it is the cultivation of clarity in thought, speech and action, through a series of effective meditation techniques handed down through the Yogic *Siddha* techniques.

One of the great *Nath Siddhas* is Patanjali, who has noted in the Yoga Sutras that the Path of Yoga consists of eight limbs, of which the first is restraint or self-discipline.

"The restraints are non-violence, truthfulness, non-stealing, sense-control, and greedlessness."

Chapter II, Sutra 30

The practiced cultivation of these *Yamas* or Restraints is a Golden Key to reaping the fruits of Happiness.

selfHealing through Postural Integration

Modern humanity has cultivated a dichotomy of body and mind. This imbalance is a major cause of ill-health. Some are drawn to cultivate their mental faculties and lose touch with their bodies. Others develop an exaggerated physique and lose touch with their mental faculties. Even when someone tries to develop both body and mind, there is isolated development and lack of integration. It is the integration of body and mind which is responsible for healing.

Asanas bring steadiness, health and lightness of limbs. A steady and pleasant postures produces mental equilibrium and prevents fickleness of mind. *Asanas* are not merely exercises: they are postures integrating body and mind. *Asanas* have been evolved over the centuries so as to exercise every muscle, nerve and gland in the body. They secure a fine physique, reduce fatigue and soothe the nerves.

When the *Asanas* are correctly combined with the breath, then they become fully effective in body-mind integration.

selfHealing by Solar Power

Our Sun is the most visible representation of Divinity for humanity. By the light of the Sun, life on Earth has originated and has blossomed. The ancient masters from time immemorial have all recognized the primacy of Solar Power for spiritual healing.

The Himalayan Masters have given humanity a series of simple, practical and effective techniques to make maximum use of the Sun's healing energy. On a physical level, the early morning and evening solar rays provide a great source of vitamin D. On an energy or *pranic* level, the Sun is the vastest reservoir and source for all life on Earth. On a spiritual level, solar practice can transform all negativity and raise the individual consciousness to a higher level.

The Solar Healing techniques combine mantra, physical movement, *Pranayama* and visualization, to provide a comprehensive system that can be practiced on its own, independent of, and augmenting any other existing spiritual practice.

Health: Chi Kung

Chi Kung describes the thousands of years old system of health and longevity, which has been practiced in China. It is based on balance and transforming the Life force. The practices utilizes gentle body movements, self-massage and breath practice to promote chi flow and meditation and harmony with earth and the cosmos. Together with a healthy, balanced diet, stress free lifestyle and harmony of body mind and spirit, longevity is assured.

The basic theory of Chi Kung Healing is that Chi in the body can be in harmony, deficiency or stagnation. If the Chi is in Harmony then health is the result. Fatigue, lack of concentration and susceptibility to disease is the result of deficiency in Chi. In stagnation, the Chi flow is blocked and pain and sickness can result. The Chi Kung exercises can be used to increase and break through Chi Stagnation with the resulting return to health.

There are many styles of Chi Kung taught, but all of them derive from the two basic schools of Taoist and Buddhist Chi Kung. Buddhist Chi Kung is related to Tantric Yoga practices brought to China, first from India and then later from Tibet. A modern exponent of Taoist Yoga is Master Mantak Chia, who has many popular books and workshops on the subject.

Health: Physical Postures "Popular Yoga"

Popular Yoga is a health maintenance system that stretches, strengthens, tones, helps to align and improves the health of the entire body. Conventional forms of exercise aims to develop specific parts of the body – abs, buns etc., or to improve cardio-vascular action.

Popular Yoga is an excellent system to promote youthfulness, fight aging and accumulation of stress and tension. It enhances body awareness with the different yoga postures stimulating and benefiting every organ.

Popular Yoga is ideal for promoting flexibility.

The use of controlled deep breathing while executing postures help to counter shortness or irregularity of breathing associated with chronic bad posture and stress.

Popular Yoga is capable of developing calmness and emotional stability.

Yoga

Yoga means union or communion. It is the union of our will with the will of the Divine. It is the union of our finite consciousness with our infinite consciousness. It is the merging of soul drop into the Ocean of Being. Yoga is composed mind unruffled. Yoga is union in *Samadhi*. Yoga is Freedom. Yoga is Self-Realization. Yoga is liberation. Yoga is Ultimate Healing.

Yoga is both a state or non-state, as well as the path towards union. Ultimately, Yoga is the cessation of the misidentification with the limited Self and with phenomena. The great Yogic scientists or Masters have taught numerous "Yogas" or Paths of Self-Realization more suitable for different temperaments than others.

Yoga is practice or *sadhana*. Just a true scientist has to perform experiments and not only rely on books, just so a Yogi has to experiment with the Self and cannot attain by relying in books.

Yoga as a path is being continuously re-invented and described according to the times and temperaments of the practitioners. It is necessary every now and then, for the Masters to present the path in various guises, without losing sight or connection to the principles laid down by the sages. The major variants are briefly described in the next pages.

Raja Yoga

This is the Royal Path, the broad highway to Being. It is generally associated with the classic Yoga Sutras by Patanjali, although it is not clear that Patanjali himself subscribed to this term, since he used the term Kriya Yoga.

This is an integrated path and is also called Ashtanga Yoga or Eightfold Yoga, because it can be described by the practice of Eight limbs. These should not be confused with consecutive steps, but are intertwined and should be viewed holistically. The Eight limbs are:

1. Self-restraints or *Yama*
2. Self-Observances or *Niyamas*
3. Postures or *Asanas*
4. Energy control or *Pranayama*
5. Internalization and Introspection or *Pratyahara*
6. Concentration or *Dharana*
7. Meditation or *Dhyana*
8. Superconsciousness or *Samadhi*

This is a path of introspection and exploration of all the heights and depths of the mind leading to transcending subconscious programs and conscious misconceptions. It is closely associated to Hatha Yoga, which is considered a ladder to Raja Yoga, focuses primarily on the first 4 of the Eight limbs.

Hatha Yoga

The word Hatha is composed of the two syllables, namely "Ha" and "tha". According to the founder of Hatha Yoga, Gorakshnath. Ha means the "moon" and tha means the "sun", and so this is the harmony of the sun and moon aspects of our being. On one level, the moon represents the mental aspects, while the sun represents the vital and physical aspects of a person. On another level, the moon represents the cooling energy flowing within a physical body, while the sun represents the hot energy which has to be harmonized for healing and health. The harmony of the mind and body results in perfect relaxation and stress relief.

The physical and energetic focus is not for the sake of physical aggrandizement but to make it a fit vessel or conduit for superconsciousness experience, the inflow of the Divine.

Hatha Yoga is very popular because it brings tangible results fairly quickly – good health, improved flexibility, strength and vitality, but should not be confused with a physical health system. The proper practice of Hatha Yoga merges into Raja Yoga.

Many of the practices of classical Hatha Yoga are extreme - physically, emotionally and mentally. Only the gentler aspects are now practiced . Even so, it is still a very powerful and forceful spiritual system that requires great courage.

Jnana Yoga

Jnana Yoga (Gyan) is commonly defined as the path of knowledge. However it is not concerned with intellectual, logical or deductive knowledge, but with Self-knowledge. Jnana Yoga is the method of union through intuitive, illuminative knowledge gained through insight meditation and some experience. It is a path of direct enquiry, without preconceptions.

This is the path only for those who are naturally inclined to absorption and self-enquiry, and is not recommended for everyone. An obsessive and obstinate personality coupled with intellectual honesty is required for success. One has to be ready to give up all beliefs, all second-hand information, all Gods and dogma. It is very difficult to believe in nothing.

A classic example in recent times of a Jnana Yoga is Ramana Maharishi who recommended the well-known enquiry : "Who Am I?"

A one-pointed mind, without distractions, without oscillating thoughts and mental disturbances is a pre-requisite. If you resonate with this path, then you can begin right now. Otherwise, alterative more active path should be practiced first. Another modern exponent of Jnana Yoga was Swami Vivekananda, who popularized Vedanta in the West.

Bhakti Yoga

The path of devotion is well-suited for those who have a strong emotional nature. It is also the most accessible to the largest number of practitioners. Bhakti is the foundation of all popular mass-appeal religious movements. It is well-developed in the Sikh religious movement of the 15th century and the Hare Krishna movement of more recent times.

The characteristic of Bhakti is a direct relationship with a deity: there are a variety of relationships depending on the personal and / or cultural inclination, including that of supplicant, friend, father, son, daughter and identity.

The practitioner will generally choose a particular aspect of the Divine, a deity or Ishtar-Deva, such as Jesus, Krishna or Ganesh, depending on his culture or attraction. By offering his love and devotion to the Ishta-Deva, the *bhakta* or devotee seeks to dissolve his ego through a progressively deeper self-surrender to the will of her God.

The characteristics of the path:

- study of the scriptures
- constant remembrance of the Deity
- unconditional self-surrender to the Lord
- dedication of all work to God
- following commandments of non-injury etc.
- expressing love to all others

Karma Yoga

This is the path of action according to the Bhagvad Gita, it is the performance of our daily work with constant awareness and at the same time without any expectation of reward. The ego or little Self is minimized by self-less action.

The results from Karma Yoga are less emotional and mental upsets – peace of mind. Tranquility. Moreover, through performance of work in the spirit of service to the Divine and for the benefit of others, salvation of the individual self is attained.

According to the Law of Karma, there is a causal relationship between action and results:

- actions performed for the benefit of others without desire for any reward are good actions and will lead one closer to the Divine
- actions performed with selfish motives or harming others are bad actions and will lead one further away from the Divine

Just as a lotus plant is not polluted by swamp water, you are not polluted by sin, if you surrender the fruits of your actions to the Divine, as you perform them.

Bhagavad Gita 5.10

Karma Yoga is seldom practiced by itself, but is incorporated in Bhakti, Hatha, Kriya, or Jnana Yogas.

Principles of Karma Yoga:

- respect for all forms of life because they are all sparks of the Divine
- look for opportunities to be of service to others. Help others in the spirit of love and compassion
- perform work for its own sake, without expectations of reward
- offer the fruits of your actions to the Divine

Do your duty to the best of your ability, O Arjuna, with your mind attached o the Lord, abandoning worry and attachment to the results. Remain calm in both success or failure. This is Karma Yoga.

Bhagavad Gita 2.48

Kundalini Yoga

Kundalini Yoga is a system focusing on the awakening of the *pranic* or psychic energy enters called *chakras*. The six main energy centers along the spine are the main concern for this path. *Kundalini* is the energy frozen at the base or 1st *chakra*, representing humanity's highest potential. The techniques of Kundalini Yoga aims to awaken the *Kundalini* energy from a potential into a kinetic state, so that it pierces all the six energy centers, resulting in the achievement of a superconsciousness. Another term for this path is Laya Yoga or the path of dissolution – the obstructions to higher consciousness are dissolved.

Tantra Yoga

Tantra is a deep and mysterious yogic path which should not be confused with the new-age sexual "tantras" which are popular in the West.

There are few genuine *tantric* masters and it needs to be emphasized that only by the power of the *Tantric Guru* who embodies the Divine Principle of Shiva can a practitioner achieve the conquest of the phenomenal world or *Samsara*.

Self-Realization is achieved through the transmutation of all negative qualities and the Self-transformation fueled by the descent of the Divine. This is the path of the razor's edge; one wrong step and you can be plunged into the delusion of desires.

The tools of *tantric* are all – encompassing – everything is great for the *tantric* will: *mantras, yantras, pranayama*, rituals, *mudras*.

Tantra Yoga has been much misunderstood both in the West and in it's country of origin India. It has played a overwhelming influence in all the spiritual aspects of India since 600 A.D. , and is still preserved in Kashmir and Bengali Tantric schools, as well as in the Tibetan Buddhist schools.

Kriya Yoga

This is simultaneous an ancient yogic path and a modern approach highly accessible to spiritual seekers. It has been popularized by Paramhansa Yogananda in the "Autobiography of a Yogi" and through an intense 30 years effort in the U.S.

Immortal Babaji has designated Kriya Yoga as the primary vehicle for spiritual evolution in these times. It is very well suited to enable a house-holder to achieve Self-realization as witnessed by its first 2 Masters, Lahiri Mahasaya and Sri Yukteswar. There should not be a misunderstanding that because Yogananda was a renunciate, that Kriya Yoga is for those who want to leave the world. Since Kriya Yoga is both action oriented, and mental, it is am advanced form of the integration of Hatha and Raja Yoga.

There are a variety of different schools, including those set up by Paramhansa Yogananda and his disciples which teaches primarily the Kriya Pranayama, or spiritual breath control and *mantras*. There are still direct disciples of Babaji, especially among the Himalayan Naths, such as Yogiraj Gurunath Siddhanath, who are initiating under his direction. When correctly practised, one round of the spiritual kriya breath is equivalent to one year of normal spiritual evolution and hence Kriya Yoga is considered to be the fastest path towards Self-Realization in our day and age.

Suggested Further Reading

Avalon, Arthur: The Serpent Power. Dove Publications. 1974. A translation of the text and commentary of *Satcakra-nirupana* [description of the six energy centers]

Feurstein, Georg: Tantra – the path of Ecstasy. Shambala, 1998.

Goswami, Shyam: Laya yoga. Inner Traditions, 1999.

Radhakrishnan, S (Tr): The Bhagavadgita. Harper Collins, 1993. Source book for many forms of yoga.

Siddhanath, Yogiraj: Wings to Freedom. Alight 2003

Shivananda, Rudra: The Yoga of Purification and Transformation. Alight Publications, 2001.

Shivananda, Rudra: In Light of Kriya Yoga. Alight 2006

Shivananda, Rudra: Insight and Guidance for Spiritual Seekers. Alight 2009

Vivekananda, Swami: Raja Yoga

Yogananda, Swami: Autobiography of a Yogi

Frequently Asked Questions

Q1. Are these energy centers real or are they only aids to meditation?

The energy centers are as real as our physical body and senses. They are more flexible and complex then we realize.

Q2. What are the *nadis*, and why haven't you talked about them in this workbook?

The *nadis* are energy channels which transport *prana* or life-energy, analogous to the blood vessels which transport blood in the physical body. The *nadis* play a critical role in the practices of Hatha and Kundalini Yogas. However, it is not necessary to consider them at an early stage of selfHealing.

Q3. I've read about these *Chakras,* but there were more of them, and the colors were different. Why?

The *Chakras* are complex and take different forms in the different bodies and levels at which a practitioner can realize. There is also the additional factor that they are susceptible to fantasies of unguided practitioners.

Even among the orthodox schools of Yoga, a variety of systems are used to effect specific results. The systems should be used together with the corresponding techniques and not mixed.

Q4. I've heard from friends that if the *Kundalini* is awakened pre-maturely, then there can be physical, emotional, and mental harm. Is there any such danger from these exercises?

The exercises that have been taught in this selfHealing workbook have been designed to be safe, and have been practiced without any harmful side-effects to a cross-section of practitioners.

It is rare that *Kundalini* is prematurely awakened. The high-profile cases which have been documented appear to be primarily caused by weakened nervous systems that were susceptible to some shock or unguided or unauthorized practices. They may appear to exhibit extraordinary experiences, skirting close to psychosis and breakdown of normal consciousness - powerful fantasies can exhibit powerful psychosomatic effects. This is not to downplay the tremendous potential that can be unleashed by the unprepared - it does happen, but not as frequently as advertised, due to the lack of competent authority and mis-diagnosis.

Q5. I've got physical problems that prevent me from performing the yoga postures. Can I still benefit from the rest of the techniques?

It is not necessary to complete all the techniques to benefit from the selfHealing program. The practice of even the first set have been found to be helpful to many.

Appendix

Additional Information on the *Chakras*

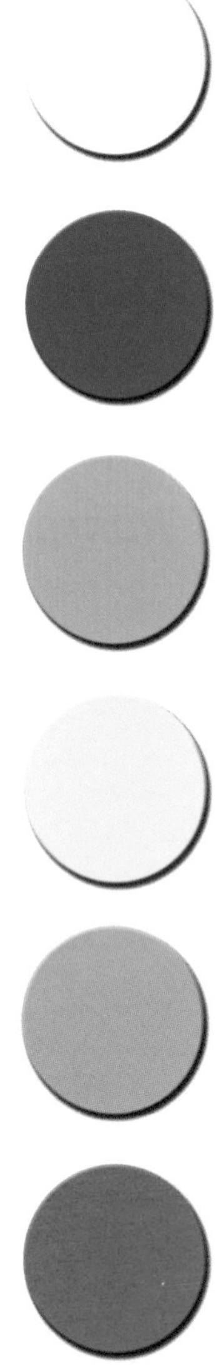

Figure 11: *Chakra* Colors

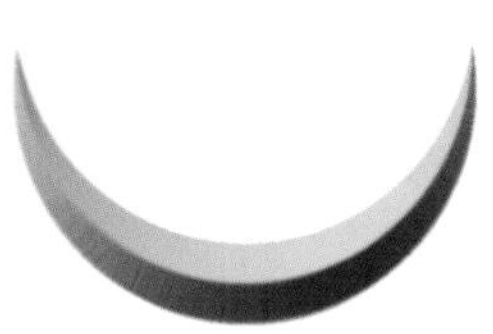

Figure 20: Earth Element **Figure 20: Water Element**

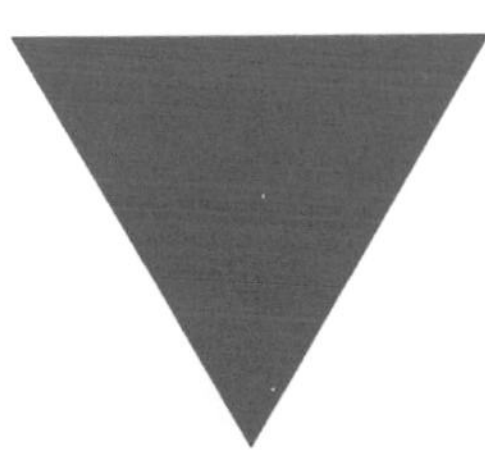

Figure 22: Fire Element **Figure 23: Air Element**

Figure 24: Space Element

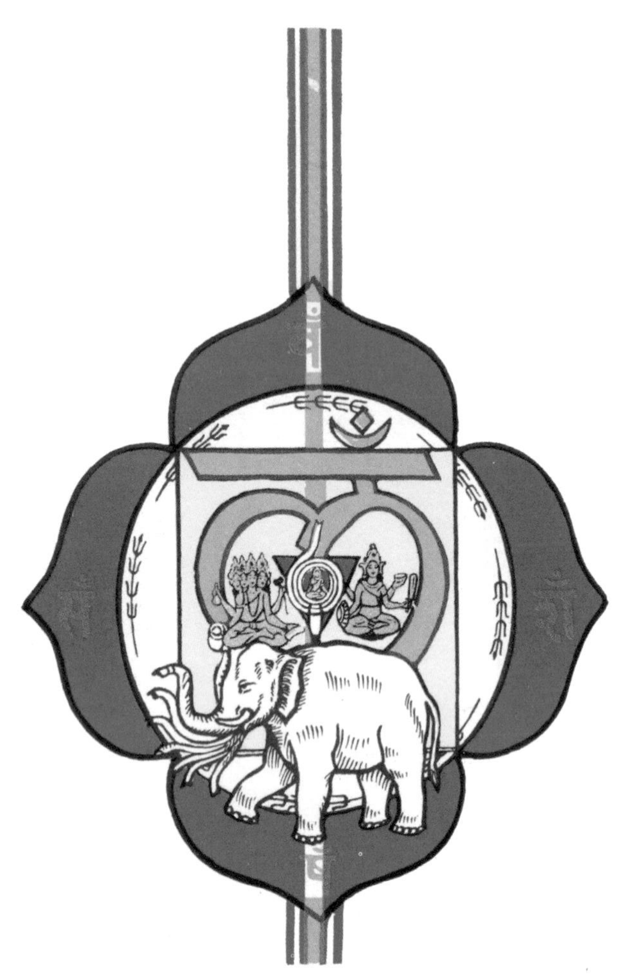

Muladhara Chakra

Verse 4

This Lotus (the Muladhara Chakra) is attached to the mouth of the Sushumna, and is placed below the genitals and above the anus. It has four petals of crimson hue. Its head hangs downward. On its petals are the four letters from Va to Sa, of the shining color of gold.

Verse 5

In this Lotus the square region of Prithivi (the earth element) surrounded by eight shining spears. It is of a shining yellow color and beautiful like lightning, as is also the Bija (the mystical "seed" syllable of the chakra, here, "Lam") of Prithivi which is within.

Verse 13

By meditating on Kundalini who shines within this chakra with the luster of ten million suns, a man becomes lord of speech, a king among men, and an adept in all kinds of learning. He becomes ever free from all diseases, and his inmost spirit becomes full of joy. Pure of disposition by his deep and musical words, he serves the foremost of the devas.

From
Sat Chakra Nirupana
of Swami Purnaananda

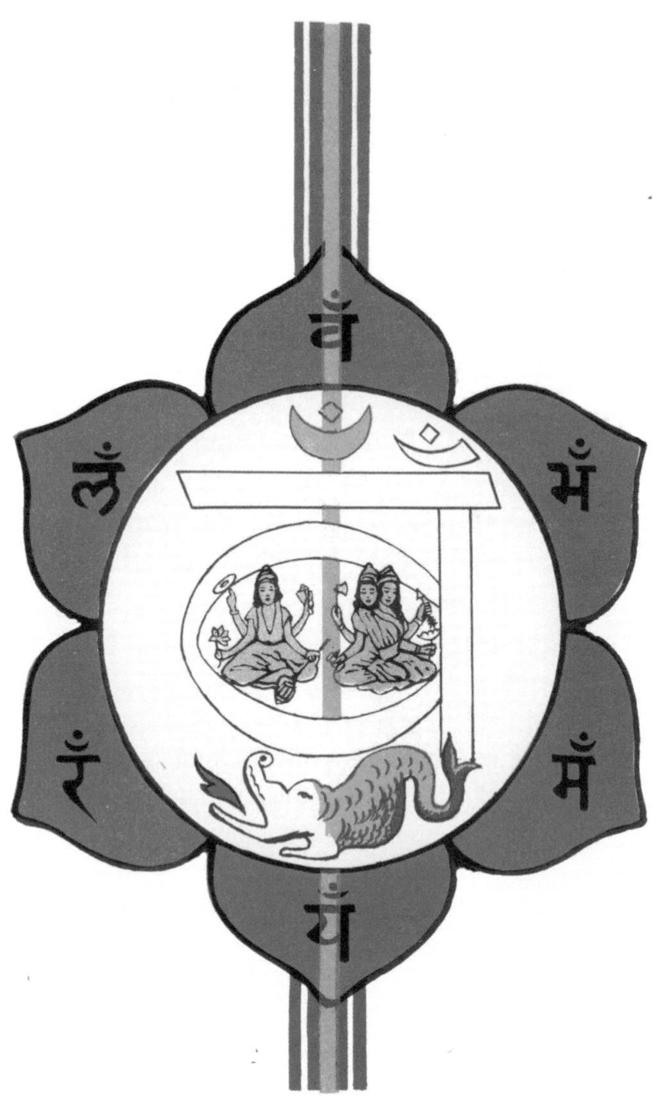

Svadhisthana Chakra

Verse 14

There is another Lotus (the Svadhisthana chakraa) placed inside the Sushumna at the root of the genitals, of a beautiful vermilion color. On its six petals are the letters from Ba to La, with the bindu (spot) superimposed over each, of the shining color of lightning.

Verse 15

Within this Lotus is the white, shining, watery region (of the god) Varuna, in the shape of a crescent, and therein, seated on a makara (a legendary animal resembling an alligator), is the bija "Vam" (connected with the principle of water, just as the bija "Lam" of the Muladhara is related to the earth element). It is stainless and white as the autumnal moon

Verse 18

He who meditates upon this stainless Lotus, which is named Svadhishtahana, is freed immediately from all his enemies such as lust, anger, greed and so forth. He becomes a lord among yogis, and is like the Sun illumining the darkness of ignorance. The wealth of his nectar-like words flows in prose and verse in well reasoned discourse.

From
Sat Chakra Nirupana
of Swami Purnaananda

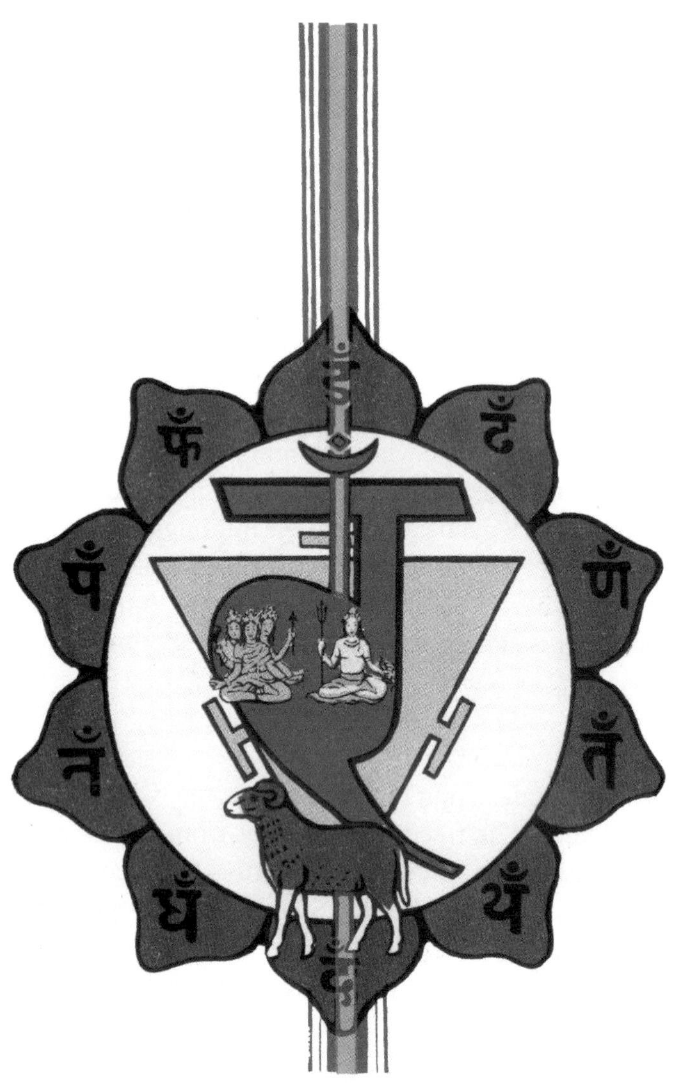

Manipura Chakra

Verse 19

Above the Svadhishthana, at the root of the navel, is a shining Lotus (Manipura Chakra) of ten petals, of the color of heavy-laden rain clouds. Within it are the sanskrit letters Da to Pha, of the color of the blue lotus with the nada and bindu above them. Meditate there on the region of Fire, triangular in form and shining like the rising sun. Outside it are three Svastika marks (one at each side of the triangle) and within it is the Bija of Vahni (the seed-mantra of Fire, "Ram")

Verse 20

Meditate upon the bija mantra seated on a ram, radiant like the rising Sun. In his lap ever dwells Rudra, who is of a pure vermilion hue. He (Rudra) is white with the ashes which he is smeared with; he is of an ancient aspect and three-eyed. His hands are placed in the attitude of granting boons and of dispelling fear. He is the destroyer of creation.

Verse 21

Here abides Lakini, the benefactress of all. She is four-armed, of radiant body, is dark of complexion, clothed in yellow raiment and decked with various ornaments, and exalted by drinking ambrosia. By meditating on this Navel Lotus the power to destroy and create (the world) is acquired. Vani (the goddess of Speech, that is, Sarasvati) with all the wealth of knowledge ever abides in the Lotus of his face (that of Fire, represented by the seed-mantra "Ram").

From
Sat Chakra Nirupana
of Swami Purnaananda

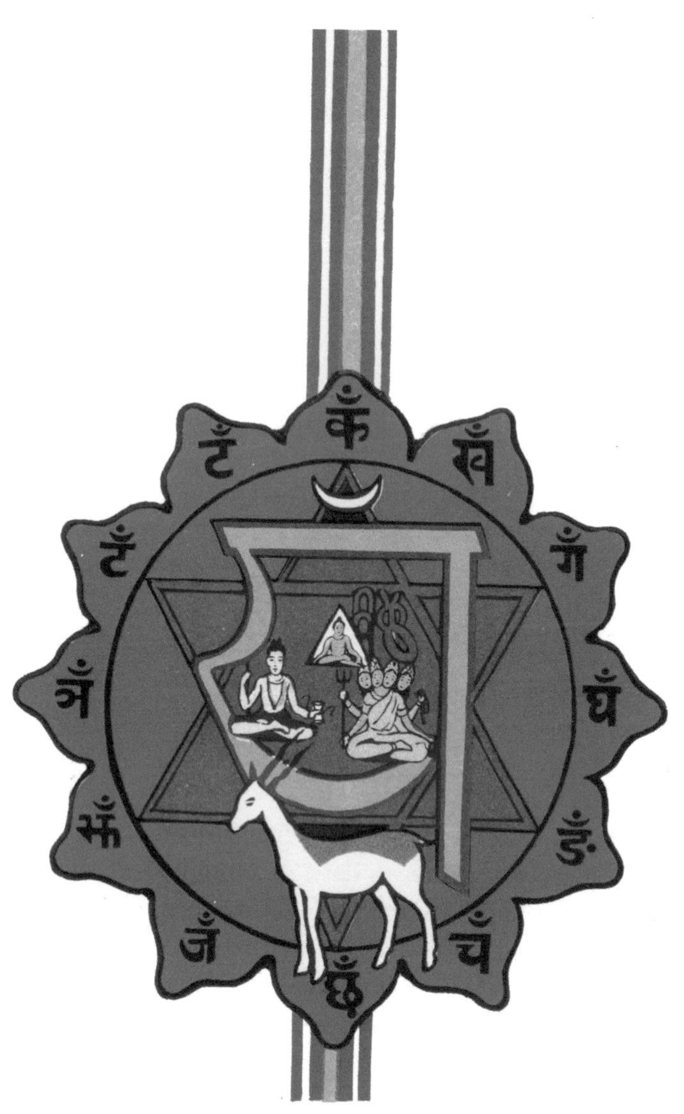

Anahata Chakra

Verse 22

Above the Manipura, in the heart, is the charming Lotus of the shining crimson color of the Bandhuka flower, with the twelve letters beginning with Ka, of the color vermilion, placed therein. It is known by its name of Anahata, and is like the celestial wishing-tree, bestowing even more than is desired. The Region of Vayu (wind), beautiful and with six corners, which is like smoke in color, is here.

Verse 23

Meditate within the region of Vayu on the sweet and excellent pavana bija (the principle of the Anahata Chakra), the bija of Vayu, “Yam”, grey as a mass of smoke, with four arms and seated on a black antelope. And within it also meditate upon the abode of Mercy, the stainless lord who is lustrous like the Sun and whose two hands make the gestures which grant boons and dispel the fears of the three worlds.

Verse 26

He who meditates on this Heart Lotus becomes like the lord of speech, and Ishvara - he is able to protect and destroy the worlds. This Lotus is like the celestial wishing tree, the abode and seat of Shiva. It is beautified by the Hamsa (here the Jivatama, the individual soul) which is like the steady tapering flame, surrounding and adorning its pericarp, illumined by the solar region.

From
Sat Chakra Nirupana
of Swami Purnaananda

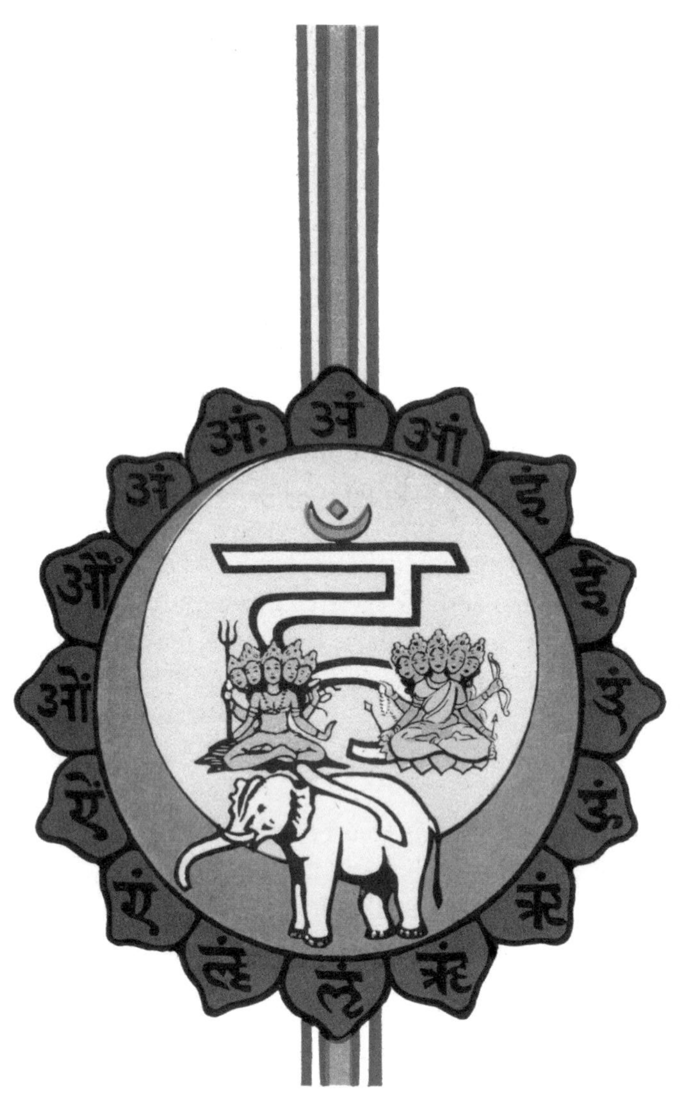

Vishuddha Chakra

Verses 28, 29

In the throat is the Lotus called the Vishuddhi which is pure and of a smoky purple hue. All the sixteen shining vowels on its sixteen petals, of a crimson hue, are distinctly visible to him whose mind is illumined. In the pericarp of this Lotus is the Ethearal Region, circular in shape and white like the full moon. On an elephant white as snow is seated the Bija of Ambara (the Ethereal Region; its bija is "Ham") who is white of color.

Of his Bija's four arms, two hold the noose and goad, and the other two make the gestures of granting boons and dispelling fear. These add to his beauty. In his lap there ever dwells the great snow-white deva, three-eyed and five-faced, with ten beautiful arms, and clothed in a tiger's skin. His body is united with that of Girija (a title of the goddess conceived as the daughter of the Mountain King), and he is known by his name Sada-shiva which signifies 'ever-beneficient.

Verse 31

He who has attained complete knowledge of the Atma (Brahman) becomes, by constantly concentrating his mind in this Lotus, a great sage, eloquent and wise, and enjoys uninterrupted peace of mind. He sees the three periods, and becomes the benefactor of all, free from disease and sorrow, and long-lived, and, like Hamsa (here, Antaratma, the true-self, that dwells by the pericarp of the Sahasrara chakra), the destroyer of endless dangers.

From
Sat Chakra Nirupana
of Swami Purnaananda

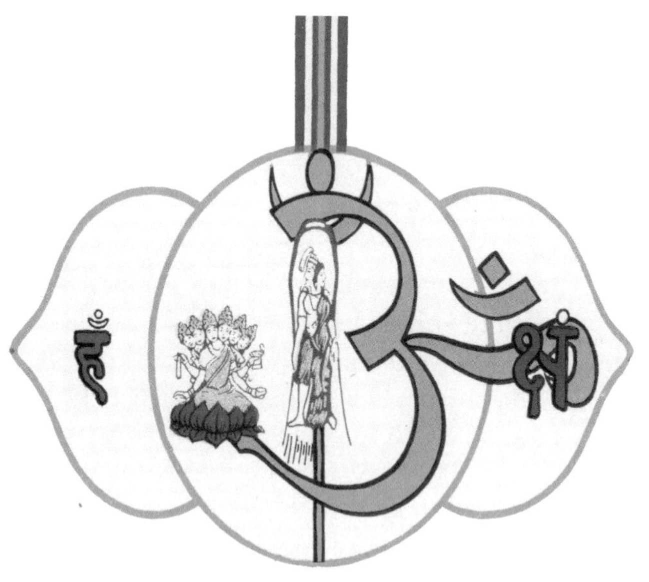

Ajna Chakra

Verse 32

The Lotus named Ajna is like the moon, beautifully white. On its two petals are the letters Ha and Ksha, which are also white and enhance its beauty. It shines with the glory of dhyana (meditation). Inside it is the Shakti Hakini, whose six faces are like so many moons. She has six arms, in one of which she holds a book (the gesture of enlightenment); two others are lifted up in gestures of dispelling fear and granting boons, and with the rest she holds a skull, a small drum, and a rosary. Her mind is pure.

Verse 33

Within this Lotus dwells the subtle mind (manas). It is well known. Inside the Yoni, the female-triangle in the pericarp is Itara Shiva. He shines like a chain of lightning flashes. The first bija of the Veda (OM), which by its luster makes visible the nadi chitrini, is also there. The sadhaka (yoga practitioner on the path to realization) with steady mind should meditate upon these accordingly.

Verse 35

Within the triangle in this Chakra ever dwells the combination of letters A and U which form the Pranava (the sacred syllable OM). It is the inner Atma as pure mind (Buddhi), and resembles a flame in its radiance.

From
Sat Chakra Nirupana
of Swami Purnaananda

The Love Power of The Heart Chakra

The Anahata Chakra or heart center is the seat of human consciousness. It is the center of transition from the animal consciousness of the three lower chakras to the divine consciousness of the higher three chakras. Most of humanity is still struggling and have their base at the navel center and often fall to the lower passionate animal consciousness of lust and fear. Those operating from the navel center are primarily concerned with controlling others and accumulating wealth and possessions. The Navel center is the seat of power, possessions and position or status.

The Heart center is the seat of that part of the soul called the prana-atma of life-force soul. The mind or manas is based at the heart center. The primary positive emotion is love and the negative emotion is hatred. It is the center where we can transform our hatred into love. It is the degree to which we have developed our capacity of love that distinguishes a true human being from an animal. It is not enough that we love our children or spouse – that is something even some higher animals can accomplish – we need to extend our love to others to whom we have no family relationship, that is to friends and eventually even to strangers.

Reacting emotionally to events, situations and relationships is the mode of the navel center and is responsible for most of the problems of humanity. If we can move our consciousness to the loving mind of the heart center, we will act and react from the perspective of love and kindness. Development of the heart center is the key to earth peace.

The heart center also rules relationships and we can see how the world is mired in relationship problems because we cannot have a relationship of equality from the navel center. The navel center is of domination and submission. One party or the other will seek to dominate. A relationship can form when one party submits but it is not human nature to submit and there cannot be lasting peace in such a lop-sided relationship despite the literary pretensions of sado-masochistic psychology. If both parties try to exert dominance, then the relationship ends abruptly. A solid foundation for a healthy relationship requires mutual respect and with both parties trying to operate from the heart center.

It is the power of awareness that can awaken the heart center. It is the awareness of love. It is the awareness of tolerance. It is the awareness of our egotistical and selfish desires. It is the awareness and willingness to look at a situation from someone else's perspective. It is awareness that can break through the barriers of the navel center and move us to the heart center.

The evolution towards higher consciousness begins when we take responsibility for seating ourselves in our loving heart center. It begins when we make the effort to act from the heart center. Peace begins when we operate from the heart center and if even a small portion of humanity activate their heart love, then there will be less and less violence and wars in this world.

1st Energy Center
Muladhara Chakra

Goal and Life Lesson
Stability & Self awareness

Location
Men: Perineum & Women: Opening of Vagina

Color
Red

Function & Sense
Survival/Physical needs & Smell

Ruling Planet, Zodiac Sign & Animal
Mars, Capricorn & Elephant

Associated Body Parts & Glands
Bones, skeletal structure & Adrenals

Oil & Crystal
Musk & Garnet

Geometric figure & Element
Yellow Square & Earth

Negative Characteristics
Materialistic, too physical, fearful, low self-esteem

Positive Characteristics
Assertive in positive manner and fearless

Possible Health Hazards
Bone Disease

2nd Energy Center
Swadhisthana Chakra

Goal and Life Lesson
Expression & Self-responsibility

Location
At the back of the spine between navel and genitals

Color
Orange

Function & Sense
Emotional balance/sexuality & Taste

Ruling Planet, Zodiac Sign & Animal
Mercury, Cancer & Fish-tailed Alligator

Associated Body Parts & Glands
Sex organs / bladder & ovaries / testes

Oil & Crystal
Sandalwood & Citrine

Geometric figure & Element
Silver Crescent & Water

Negative Characteristics
Erratic emotionality, driven by guilt, inability to face reality

Positive Characteristics
Creativity, harmony between feelings and expression

Possible Health Hazards
Lower back problems, frigidity or impotence

3rd Energy Center
Manipura Chakra

Goal and Life Lesson
Effectiveness & Self-esteem/self-respect

Location
Behind the navel at the spine

Color
Yellow

Function & Sense
Will-power & Sight

Ruling Planet, Zodiac Sign & Animal
Sun, Leo & Ram

Associated Body Parts & Glands
Digestive system, muscles & Pancreas

Oil & Crystal
Cinnamon and Topaz

Geometric figure & Element
Red downward-facing triangle & Fire

Negative Characteristics
"Bossiness", Anger, Judgemental

Positive Characteristics
Energetic, Gentle

Possible Health Hazards
Digestive problems and diabetes

4th Energy Center
Anahata Chakra

Goal and Life Lesson
Love, Compassion & Self-acceptance

Location
At the spine opposite the center of chest

Color
Green

Function & Sense
Relationship & Touch

Ruling Planet, Zodiac Sign & Animal
Venus, Taurus & Antelope

Associated Body Parts & Glands
Hearts, Lungs, circulation & Thymus

Oil & Crystal
Rose & Emerald

Geometric figure & Element
Smoky-green interlaced Triangle

Negative Characteristics
Self-pity, possessiveness

Positive Characteristics
Unconditional love

Possible Health Hazards
High blood pressure, tendency towards heart disease

5th Energy Center
Vishuddha Chakra

Goal and Life Lesson
Harmony & Self-expression

Location
Throat

Color
Blue

Function & Sense
Communication & Hearing

Ruling Planet, Zodiac Sign & Animal
Jupiter, Sagittarius & Bull

Associated Body Parts & Glands
Mouth, throat, ears & Thyroid / Parathyroid

Oil & Crystal
Myrrh & Lapis Lazuli / Blue Sapphire

Geometric figure & Element
Blue Circle & Space

Negative Characteristics
Arrogance, Emotional blockage

Positive Characteristics
Inspired communication

Possible Health Hazards
Sore throat, thyroid problems

6th Energy Center
Ajna Chakra

Goal and Life Lesson
Wisdom and Self-knowledge

Location
Third-eye (in the brain: third ventricle)

Color
Indigo

Function & Sense
Wisdom & Intuitive vision

Ruling Planet, Zodiac Sign & Animal
Saturn, Capricorn & Hamsa Swan

Associated Body Parts & Glands
Eyes, base of skull & Pituitary gland

Oil & Crystal
Rose Germanium & Amethyst

Element
Mind

Negative Characteristics
Too analytical and dogmatic

Positive Characteristics
Charismatic, highly intuitive, visionary

Possible Health Hazards
Headaches, nervous disorders

7th Energy Center
Sahasrara Chakra

Goal and Life Lesson
Truth and Self-realization

Location
Crown

Color
Violet and white

Function & Sense
Spirituality & Divinity

Ruling Planet, Zodiac Sign
Ketu, Aquarius

Associated Body Parts & Glands
Brain cortex, skin & Pineal gland

Oil & Crystal
Lavender & clear quartz

Element
Thought

Negative Characteristics
Depression, psychosis

Positive Characteristics
Magnetic personality, peace and transcendence

Possible Health Hazards
Bone Disease